F. R. (Frederick Ransom) Campbell

The Language of Medicine

A Manual Giving the Origin, Etymology, Pronunciation, And Meaning of the

Technical Terms Found in Medical Literature

F. R. (Frederick Ransom) Campbell

The Language of Medicine
A Manual Giving the Origin, Etymology, Pronunciation, And Meaning of the Technical Terms
Found in Medical Literature

ISBN/EAN: 9783744645911

Printed in Europe, USA, Canada, Australia, Japan

Cover: Foto ©Andreas Hilbeck / pixelio.de

More available books at **www.hansebooks.com**

THE LANGUAGE OF

MEDICINE

A MANUAL GIVING THE ORIGIN,
ETYMOLOGY, PRONUNCIATION, AND MEANING OF
THE TECHNICAL TERMS FOUND IN
MEDICAL LITERATURE

BY

F. R. CAMPBELL, A. M., M. D.

PROFESSOR OF MATERIA MEDICA AND THERAPEUTICS,
MEDICAL DEPARTMENT OF NIAGARA UNIVERSITY

NEW YORK
D. APPLETON AND COMPANY
1888

PREFACE.

THE object of this work is to provide the medical student with a suitable means of acquiring the vocabulary of his science. Like Shakespeare, the great majority of medical students have but "small Latine and lesse Greeke." Even those who have enjoyed the advantages of literary colleges are often unable to apply their knowledge of the classical languages in determining the etymology and meaning of ordinary medical words, partly because the classics are studied more from a literary than a philological point of view, but largely because the words most used in medical works seldom appear in the Latin and Greek with which tney are familiar.

In studying mathematics or grammar the pupil begins with definitions of the new words to be employed. In medicine, also, much valuable time could be saved if the student would first master the meaning of the technical terms by which the principles of the science are to be carried into his mind. The words must be understood before thoughts which they convey can be comprehended. In the first part of this work are discussed many of the elementary principles of philology and etymology, illustrated by common words occurring in medical literature. Coleridge has said that we may often derive more useful knowledge from the history of a word than from the history of a campaign. In medicine we may often obtain more practical benefit from the study of some word with an account of the errors involved therein, than from the study of a new theory which rises like a balloon only to burst like a bubble. A brief history of medicine, from a linguistic point of view, is given in order that the sources of our technical words may be known.

In part second will be found the majority of the Latin words used in medical works. The principles of Latin grammar which are employed in nomenclature and prescription writing are discussed and exercises for translation are given in order that the student may fix the words and grammatical principles in his mind.

The subject of orthoepy is incidentally discussed and a list of many words commonly mispronounced is given. The majority of these have been collected in the class-room, but many, very many, have been mispronounced by medical society orators and college professors who have persisted in propagating their orthoepical blunders through the medical profession until one hesitates before pronouncing some words correctly for fear of being misunderstood.

In part third will be found the principal words of Greek origin with a description of the method of converting Greek words into Latin and English. In part fourth are collected the majority of the words transferred from the modern foreign languages into our medical vocabulary. In determining the correct etymology of words the author has, in the main, followed Curtius, Skeat, and Halsey. But philologists, like doctors, sometimes disagree, and in these cases the writer has selected what appeared to him the most reasonable derivation.

It may be urged that this work should have been undertaken by a professor of the languages rather than by a physician. But the teacher of languages knows comparatively little of the real needs and defects of the average medical student, while a physician reasonably familiar with the ancient and modern languages is able to apply his linguistic knowledge in

PREFACE.

a manner at once more interesting and instructive to the medical student.

In conclusion, the author must acknowledge his indebtedness to the following authors, for without their aid the preparation of this book would have been an impossibility: —

ANDREWS, *Latin-English Lexicon.*
BIONDELLI, *Studii Linguistici.*
BRACHET, *Dictionaire Etymologique de la Langue Francaise*
CURTIUS, *Grundzuege der Griechischen Etymologie.*
DARMESTETER, *Life of Words as the Symbols of Ideas.*
Encyclopædia Britannica.
FARRAR, *Origin of Language.*
HALSEY, *Etymology of Latin and Greek.*
LIDDELL and SCOTT, *Greek-English Lexicon.*
DR. MEREDITH, *Errors of Speech.*
PAREIRA, *Physicians' Prescription Book.*
SKEAT, *Etymological English Dictionary.*
THOMAS, *Medical Dictionary.*
TRENCH, *On the Study of Words.*
WHITNEY, *Language and the Study of Language.*

FREDERICK R. CAMPBELL.

BUFFALO, N. Y., *January, 1888.*

CONTENTS.

PART I.

ORIGIN OF THE LANGUAGE OF MEDICINE.

PART II.

THE LATIN ELEMENT IN THE LANGUAGE OF MEDICINE.

ORIGIN OF THE LANGUAGE OF MEDICINE.

CHAPTER I.

INTRODUCTION.

SCIENCES and arts, like nations, have languages of their own. When a nation makes progress in civilization, new words are formed to express new thoughts and discoveries. When old institutions die out, the words used to symbolize them disappear. So it is with the language of a science ; with each new theory or discovery a new word is born; with each exploded hypothesis or abandoned instrument an old word dies. Words in a language like the cells of an animal are constantly forming and dying, this process being one of the surest indications of life. To use the words of a poet :—

> " Life itself is but a rider
> On the myriad steeds of death,
> Since some tissue, some secretion
> Lives and dies at every breath.
> But the force which binds the atoms,
> Which controls secreting glands,
> Is the same that guides the planets
> Acting by divine commands."

Nations disappear from the political map of the world and we often speak of them and their languages as " dead ; " but their life is not really gone, for their blood is mingled with that of their conquerors and the words used to designate truths discovered by them are retained as monuments, to tell the story of their customs and civilization. There is no longer a Roman empire but Latin is the basis of the languages of five great nations and has exerted a lasting influence upon the vocabularies of every civilized race. The so-called sciences of alchemy and astrology have long slept in the dim and dusty past, but many of the terms employed by their devotees still exist in scientific nomenclature.

Many of these words have assumed meanings entirely different from the original. *Al cksir*, elixir, with the alchymists meant, the philosopher's stone, but is now applied to an agreeable preparation of a medicine. So also many words which arose from strange medical notions, long ago abandoned, still remain in our language with their forms and significations more or less changed. *Mania*, Greek μανία, or μῆνις as used by Homer, is derived from the same root as μήν, the moon, and meant originally, the moon sickness, being the exact counterpart of the Latin *lunaticus* from *luna*, the moon. These words are still employed to designate states of mental aberration although we ridicule the aetiological notions involved in them.

A careful study of the etymology of medical terms would enable us to reconstruct, in a measure, the history of our art, just as the geologist from strata and fossils, tells the story of the earth's creation and the development of all the life it now contains. By examining the silt at the mouth of a river we can determine the character of the soil through which the waters have passed; so also we can discover in the ancient medical words which have drifted down through the ages, indications of the sources of our knowledge, of our past errors and successes. We still talk of *plagues*, a word derived from πληγή, a blow inflicted by the almighty gods to wreak vengeance upon guilty mortals; of *melancholy* from μέλας black and χόλη bile, which was supposed to cause this affection; of *poultices* which are no longer bean puddings or porridge, πόλτος; of *arteries*, from ἀρτηρία a wind pipe or air tube, because they were supposed to contain nothing but air; and yet the original ideas represented by these words have long since faded from our view. In fact, as Archbishop Trench has shown, we find poetry, history and ethics in words, even in medical terms, which are supposed by those ignorant of their history, to be the symbols of the dryest of facts and ideas.

Saturn, one of the gods of the older school, has come down to us in *saturnine* poisoning; Mars, the god of war and iron weapons, has given us the *martial* preparations; Jupiter Ammon, the horned god, is remembered in *ammonia*, hartshorn; some of our instruments are of *Vulcanized* rubber; Mercury, as a Roman, has presented us with *mercurial* preparations, as a Greek with name of Hermes, ("Ερμῆς) he sees that our tubes are *hermetically* sealed. Venus, as a Roman, has a particular portion of the female anatomy, the *mons veneris*, dedicated to her memory, while she has sent us a host of diseases, the venereal, which are very remunerative to the doctor but not very complimentary to herself. As a Greek goddess with the name of Aphrodite, (Ἀφροδίτη) we see her in the class of *aphrodisiac* remedies. Eros ("Ηρως), the Greek Cupid is remembered in *Erotomania*, Psyche (Ψυχή) his companion in *psychiatry*, and from Iris, the messenger of the gods, we now extract a cholagogue. All Olympus thus seems to have been interested in medicine, while demigods, nymphs, satyrs, and naiads stroll through the various branches of our science giving their names, here to a plant used medicinally, and there to a disease, symptom, or part of the body.

When we speak of the *tendo Achillis* we are reminded of that classical tale relating how the son of Peleus was held by the heel and dipped by his seaborn mother into the river Styx to make him invulnerable; how this particular tendon and the parts about it were not immersed, and how Paris succeeded in inflicting a mortal wound in this locality. There is poetry too in the names of drugs and plants. *Phosphorus* (φῶς light φέρω to carry), is the morning star, the light bearer; *Cypripedium* in Venus's slipper, from *Cypris* one of her names; while *morphine* recalls *Morpheus*, the changing god of dreams, who lulled mankind to sleep.

Even the names of diseases, strange as it may seem, contain metaphors and other poetical figures. *Carbuncles* are like the purple reddish gems of the same name, *icterus* (Greek ʼίκτερος) is the name of the yellow bird, while *iliac passion* is a phrase which recalls the spear thrust and the tragic sufferings on the Cross. History is found everywhere illustrated in words, *calculate* and *testify* take us back to the days when men told members with pebbles, *calculi*, and cast their votes with shells, *testae*. *Gentianus* of Illyria is said to have discovered the virtues of the plant named after him. *Magnets* were first known in Magnesia, chalk, *creta*, in Crete.

We all know what *cretinism* is, yet few are aware that *cretin* and *Christian* were originally the same word. The Arian refugees of the Pyrinees were anciently called *Christaas*, in French *Chreticns* or Christians. Long residence in the dim valleys with frequent intermarriages of blood relations in time developed a peculiar form of idiocy associated with enlargement of the thyroid gland. People afflicted with this malady are still called Christians under the name *cretins*, while *cretinism* means etymologically Christianity.

Idiocy also has a historical origin. The ancient Athenians were a nation of politicians. Those who did not hold office were designated as ἰδιῶται, private citizens, to distinguish them from the office holders. In time a man who was not a public servant and had never had an opportunity to serve the state as such, was looked upon as a person of very inferior mental capacity, and finally *idiocy* assumed a meaning among the Ancient Greeks quite similar to that which we now assign to it.

There is in mankind a tendency to call impure things by better names than they deserve. This custom, called *euphemism* is frequently illustrated in medical nomenclature, and we find the names pagan divinities who once tuned the harps of poets and inspired the genius of artists, applied to parts or functions of the body whose vulgar names we would be ashamed to write. Venus in our art is not the goddess of love, but of lust, Priapus has nothing to do with the fertility of gardens, but is distinguished only for his enormous *membrum virile* in a constant state of erection; satyrs and nymphs no longer sport by babbling brooks on vineclad hills, revelling in choral dances with Pan and Bacchus, but are famed only for their salacity, and Hymen, the god of marriage and of nuptial songs is remembered only by a delicate female membrane supposed to be ruptured on the wedding night.

When we recall the numerous allusions in our science to the heathen deities of old, the "sacred disease," *epilepsy*, the "sacred fire," *erysipelas*, the "sacred muscle," *transversalis lumborum*, and the "sacred bone," *os sacrum*, we feel that our art is still redolent with the paganism and superstitions of antiquity. When we think of "St. Anthony's fire," "St. Vitus' dance," and St. Ignatius' bean, we wander to mediaeval shrines more pious but not less superstitious. But with all these relics of vagaries and past errors, our science is still advancing to a higher plain, and the day may come when the comma bacillus, the gonococcus, and many other terms will likewise be classed among words marking the delusions of the past; for many a hypothesis supported by the ablest of physicians, has disappeared from the pages of our medical books leaving only a few words, like fossils, to tell future generations the story of their rise and fall.

CHAPTER II.

The Historical Sources of the Language of Medicine.

IN tracing the history of the English language we learn that the earliest known inhabitants of Britain were the Celts whose language has left but few traces in our vernacular. Then came the Saxons, sweeping all before them and forcing their vocabulary upon the original inhabitants who were not destroyed or driven into the mountain fastnesses. A few centuries later the Normans conquered the Saxons, and, although they could not abolish the vocabulary of these Teutons, they forced many words upon them, and the language of England became a Normanized Saxon. The Christian Church, with its Latin tongue, and the revival of Greek learning, in their turn brought many erudite terms from these sources into the English language, while the Crusades, commerce, and Continental wars have introduced many more foreign terms, making the English language what it is to-day.

In a similar manner we may trace the developmental history of the language of medicine, which, like the language of a nation, has a story and a dictionary of its own. The art of medicine was born with the Aryan race, but the language of the Aryans, like that of the Celts, has had only an indirect influence upon the subsequent vocabularies. The Greeks cultivated medical science until it attained a high degree of development; then, as the Normans conquered the Saxons, so the Romans conquered the Greeks, and the language of medicine became a·Latinized Greek, as, in the former

2

case, it became a Normanized Saxon. For half a mil-
lennium in the middle ages the true science of medicine
dwelt with the Arabs, and when it came back to Latin-
speaking countries it brought some Moorish words and
notions in its train. Then, when Greek learning was
revived in the fifteenth century, many of the older terms,
which had been lost, were again restored, and Greek has
remained the favorite source from which we derive
medical terms at the present day, although, of late, many
words from various modern languages, especially the
French, have found their way into our medical literature.

We will now discuss the sources of our medical
terms in a more detailed manner.

An eminent comparative philologist has devoted
considerable attention to the language and civilization of
the primitive Aryans. Although there are no written
specimens of their tongue, and no tabulated history of
their nation, he has been able to gather a great deal of
interesting information from the roots of Aryan words
found in other languages, thus reconstructing their
vocabulary and grammar, much as the geologist, from a
single fossil bone, will picture to you the antediluvian
animal of which it formed a part. He thus discovers
that this ancient people rode in carts drawn by oxen,
wore clothes made of wool, had a religion with a priesthood, and employed physicians.

Sanskrit, the sacred language of the Hindoos,
is the elder brother of the Indo-European linguistic
family, and of this we possess some very ancient
books on medicine and other sciences. Long before
the days of Homer, at least a thousand years before
Christ, these Hindoos possessed a knowledge of
medicine which was not surpassed by that of the
Greeks in the days of Hippocrates. The *Ayur Veda,*

with the commentaries of *Charaka* and *Susruta*, were probably in existence at that early date, and there is considerable evidence that the *Ayur Veda*, the oldest medical treatise in the world, is an abridgement of a still older and larger work. The dignity and ethics of the medical profession of that ancient race have never been surpassed. Before the young Brahmin was allowed to study medicine, he must pass a special examination in regard to his moral and intellectual attainments. In his final examination, so various and extensive were the qualifications desired, that, it is said, "they were never found combined in a single mortal on earth, and but rarely in heaven." There were laws enforced by the Rajah regulating the practice of medicine and the suppression of quackery. "The charlatan may be known," says Susruta, "by his vanity and his ill-will toward the good physician. He flatters the patient's friends, takes reduced fees, is hesitating and doubtful in performing difficult operations, and pretends that his want of success is caused by bad attendants. Such persons avoid the society of the learned physician as they would a jungle." *

The ancient Hindoo physician was familiar with practical anatomy. All the larger viscera of the body were known and named. Susruta says: "A holy man (physician-priest) should dissect, in order that he may know the internal structure of the body." He also gives minute directions for the selection of a subject. Seven kinds of joints were known and described, nerves were distinguished from tendons, and the different layers of the skin had been discovered. Pathology, like that of the Greeks at a later period, was based upon humors. Indeed, this humoral pathology remained in medical science until the last century, and traces of it still exist

---

* Dr. H. T. Wise, "History of Medicine," Vol. I.

in our language. "Salt rheum," from ῥεῦμα, a humor,
is a common expression with the laity. What does it
mean? Merely that there is a salty humor in the blood.
Rheumatism meant, originally, to be full of humors, from
the Greek ῥευματίζω. The proper mixture of the humors
produced temperaments, from *tempero*, to season or
restrain. Thus there are bilious, lymphatic, sanguine
and mixed temperaments, depending upon the prepon-
derating humor. When we say that a horse has the
distemper, we mean, literally, that the equilibrium of
humors has been impaired.

So much for this diversion from our subject.
In materia medica the Hindoos had made great
discoveries. The properties of many plants were
known; leeches were used; common salt, borax, sulphur, four kinds of mercury, antimony, zinc, iron and
arsenic were all administered in a remarkably intelligent
manner. Surgery was also highly developed. Susruta
gives directions for performing lithotomy, laparotomy,
hysterotomy, and various autoplastic operations, particularly rhinoplasty. Physicians from India traveled through
the world performing operations and attending the sick.
It is probable, though not certain, that they visited
Greece, and it may be that the lithotomists whom Hippocrates mentions as being the only ones who should per-
form the operation for removing stone, were Indians, and
far better surgeons than the Father of Medicine himself.
We know that when, shortly after the death of Hippocrates, Alexander the Great invaded Asia, Indian physicians possessed of wonderful skill, even being able to
raise the dead, were mentioned by Arrian. It is also
claimed that many of the Hippocratic treatises are mere
translations of Hindoo works. In scarcely any other
way can we account for the remarkable knowledge of

anatomy displayed by the Greeks at this time, for we
know that practical anatomy was unknown to Hippocrates. Another evidence that Greek medicine was
indebted to that of the Hindoos may be deduced from
the fact that many drugs employed by the Greeks have
Hellenized Sanskrit names. The following may be
mentioned:

GREEK.	SANSKRIT.	LATIN.	ENGLISH.
Καστόριον	*kasturi*	castor	musk
Κάστανα	fr. *kasta* testicle and chestnut	castanea	chestnut
Κάρδαμον	*ciradamun* cira a pod	cardamomum	cardamom
Κάνναβις	*cana*	cannabis	hemp
Μακήρ	*makura*	macis	mace
Μόσχος	*muschka* testicle	moschus	musk
Πέπερι	*pippali*	piper	pepper
Σάνταλον	*candana* shining	santalum	sandal wood
Σάκχαρον	*carkara*	saccharum	sugar
Ζιγγιβερίς	*gringavera:* antler shaped	zingiber	ginger

Some anatomical names, also, are either taken directly
from the Sanskrit or, what is more probable, both the
Sanskrit and the Greek are derived from the primitive
Aryan. Examples :—

SANSKRIT.	GREEK.	LATIN.	ENGLISH.
Ciras	κάρα	caput	head, kopf *Germ.*
Hrid	καρδία	cor	heart
Naurce	νεῦρον	nervus	nerve
Medhara	μυελός	medulla	marrow
Osthi	ὀστέον	os	bone
Pitta bile	πιτύιτα	pituita	spittle
Vasti	κύστις	vesica	bladder

Some words have found their way into Latin and
English from the Sanskrit which are not observed in the
Greek. For example *sulphur*, often spelled *sulfur*, is

from the Sanskrit *culvari*. In Greek the word for sulphur is θεῖον *divine*, because it was supposed to have a
purifying power, prophetic of its use as a disinfectant on
earth and in Hades.   This Greek word appears in the
nomenclature of the sulphur compounds, dithionic,
bisulphuric, trithionic, etc.

The student will observe that these words change
form in passing from one language to another, just as
many of the lower animal and vegetable organisms
undergo morphological changes when the medium which
surrounds them is altered.   On this account it is very
difficult to trace many words to their birthplace, and our
knowledge of the influence of Hindoo medicine upon
that of the Greeks is very obscure.   We may state, however, that the art, much more than the language of
medicine, was affected by Eastern influence.

The same may be said of Egyptian medicine in regard
to its influence upon the Greek.   We know that many
Greeks visited Egypt and studied their sciences.   Indeed, it
was the custom with historians, at one time, to derive all
the sciences from Egypt.   Yet, with the possible exception
of πύραμις, pyramid, and the names of a few divinities,
there are scarcely any Egyptian words to be found in
the Greek language.   The Egyptians were famed for
their specialties.   Herodotus tells us that they had " one
physician for the eyes, another for the head, and another
for the parts about the belly."   They were the first
dentists of whom we have any knowledge, for false teeth
and gold fillings have been found in the mouths of
mummies.   They were able to operate for cataract suc-
cessfully, could remove stone from the bladder, knowing
both the supra-pubic and perinæal operation, and yet,
with all their skill and all their intercourse with Greece,
few, if any, Egyptian words found their way into the

vocabularies of medical writers.   The Greeks prided themselves upon the purity of their language, regarding all foreign words as barbarisms, and, accordingly, avoided the importation of words to represent the ideas acquired abroad.

The Greek element is the foundation of the language of medicine, and it is of great importance that the scientific student should know at least the first principles of this tongue.   In the works of Homer, who is supposed to have lived some 900 years before Christ, we find frequent references to the healing art.   There were no surgeons who devoted themselves especially to that branch of practice.   Podalirius and Machaon, the sons of Æsculapius, were called ἰατροί, or ἄνδρες ἰατροί, *healing men*, but they fought in the ranks like the other heroes, and there are many instances in which other leaders extracted darts and applied styptic herbs to the wounds. The word ἰατρός is derived from ἰάομαι, to heal, and is always used by Homer for surgeon, there being no evidence that medicines (φάρμακα) were given internally. The word ἰατρός, or ἰατρία, healing, curing, is preserved in the technical terms *psychiatry*, mind healing, the cure of mental diseases, and in *pædiatry*, child healing, the treatment of children's diseases, derived from ψυχή, the mind, and παῖς, a child, respectively.   The *pharmaca* were always of a vegetable nature, and were styptic and anodyne in their action.   The word χειρουργός is of later origin, and means, literally, *hand work*, from χείρ, the hand, and ἔργον, work; whence we have χειρουργία, handiwork, Latin *chirurgia*, a word which, with slight modification, means *surgery* in nearly all modern languages; thus, in Italian and Spanish *cirugia*, German and French *chirurgie*, Old English *chirurgery*; whence the modern form, *surgery*.   When men became afflicted with non-

surgical affections, the disease was looked upon as a
punishment sent by the gods, just as our Western
Indians, and some other people not so barbarous but
quite as superstitious, regard bodily disorders at the
present day. When the pestilence (λοιμός, from which
our word loimology is derived) appeared among the
Grecian hosts at Troy, it was explained by the anger of
Apollo, who was wreaking vengeance upon the offenders:

> " He came as comes the night. At first he smote
> The mules and the swift dogs, and then on man
> He turned his deadly arrows, while all around
> Glared evermore the frequent funeral pyres."

In this case the Greeks did not imitate Asa, of Old
Testament fame, who " sought not to the Lord in his
affliction, but to the physicians," and, as a consequence,
" slept with his fathers." But neglecting Podalirius and
Machaon, they piously consulted the priest of Apollo, to
help them appease the anger of the infuriated god. He
ordered a general ablution of the Greek army—very
good advice in its way—and a sacrifice of a hundred
oxen, and soon the pestilence disappeared. The word
physician comes indirectly from the Greek through the
Latin *physicianus*. The Greek φυσικός means pertaining
to nature or growth (φύσις). From this our words *physic*,
physics, and many others are derived. The φυσικοί,
physici, were not physicians as the word is understood
to-day, but natural scientists; and as these scientists
understood medicine, the science most appreciated by
the people, the word finally came to be applied to
medical practitioners alone. During the early centuries
of our era the *physici* were sorcerers, and *physic*, τὰ φυσικά,
meant drugs of magical origin.

The Homeric surgeons had no knowledge of anatomy except such as was acquired from the treatment of

wounds and the evisceration of animals, as was practiced in making sacrifices. All the external parts of the body and the principal internal organs were known and named, the words employed by Homer being found in scientific medical works at the present day.*

But the true science of medicine, as we now understand it, came into existence with Hippocrates, who lived 460–377 B. C. With the exception of an accurate knowledge of osteology, Hippocrates was not much more intimately acquainted with anatomy than were the Homeric heroes. He mentions, with considerable satisfaction, the existence of a human skeleton in one of the temples of Æsculapius, and it was from this source that his accurate knowledge of bones was derived. To him, muscles were but flesh, and veins ($\varphi\lambda\acute{\epsilon}\beta\epsilon\varsigma$) were only *gushers* (from $\varphi\lambda\acute{\epsilon}\omega$, to gush, *cf.* the Latin *fleo* to weep). The word *artery* ($\dot{a}\rho\tau\eta\rho\dot{\iota}a$) is restricted to the windpipe, while $\nu\epsilon\ddot{\upsilon}\rho a$ (*neura*), in the Hippocratic age, represented both nerves and tendons. The brain was a gland secreting mucus; the heart, a muscle containing four cavities, two for the reception of air, and two fountains of life; the lungs were for the reception of air to cool the internal fires.

But the Hippocratic descriptions of diseases and symptoms are quite accurate. He was a true artist in portraying the signs and symptoms of disease. The

---

* The following medical words are found in the Iliad and Odyssey, with meanings identical with those of the present day: Carpus, chole, cleido, coma, corona, crocus, cranium, cyanic, cystis, encephalon, entera, hidrosis, ischium, omphalus, ophthalmos, omo-, picric, phrenic, phyton, phthisis, splanchna, sternum, stethos, and syringe.

Besides these, there are many words which are similar in form in Homeric Greek and in modern medical works, but have different meanings. The following may be taken as examples: Æther, amnion, amœba, astragalus, clonos, corymb, didymi, ephialtes, gastro-, iris, ichor, melissa, mesodme, meconium, molybdenum, narcosis, nymphæ, pleura, phial, phlebs, phalanges, sponge, trachea and troche.

Hippocratic countenance, *facies Hippocratica*,* has become a classical phrase. The names given by him to diseases, in many instances, remain in the nosologies of the present day, and his method of forming words to represent pathological processes has served as a model for all succeeding generations.

The next great name which has had a lasting influence upon the language of medicine is that of Aristotle, who was born 384 B. C.   He was the inventor of comparative anatomy.   His classification of animals, based upon anatomical peculiarities, was so excellent that Cuvier, more than 2,000 years afterward, found no occasion to seek a better.   Aristotle gives the first reliable description of the brain, and the word *aorta* (ἀορτή, from ἀείρω, to rise up) was probably invented by him.   He was familiar with the whole alimentary canal and the surrounding viscera.   He divides the intestines into parts quite similar to those described in modern works, the terms now used being, in many cases, mere translations of the Greek words used by Aristotle.

The foundation of the Alexandrian Library by the Greeks of Egypt, 380 B. C. and the legalization of human dissection gave a new impetus to the study of anatomy and physiology, and a few years later we observe the names of Erasistratus and Herophilus, the first Greek anatomists.   Erasistratus described the valves of the heart, the cranial nerves, and perhaps distinguished motor from sensory nerves.   Herophilus whose name is

---

* A sharp nose, hollow eyes, collapsed temples ; the ears cold, contracted, and their lobes turned out ; the skin about the forehead being rough, distended and parched ; the color of the whole face being green, black, livid or lead-colored.—*Hippocrates' Prognostics.*

Shakespeare, in describing the death of Falstaff, seems to have been familiar with this description of the *facies Hippocratica :* "For after I saw him fumble with the sheets, and play with flowers, and smile upon his fingers' ends, I knew there was but one way ; for his nose was as sharp as a pin, and he babbled of green fields, So he bade me lay more clothes on his feet ; I put my hands into the bed and felt them, and they were as cold as any stone."—*Henry V., II., 3.*

commemorated in *torcular Herophili*, the wine press of Herophilus, was the first vivisectionist, and was even accused of vivisecting condemned criminals. He gave the names to the *choroid plexus* and *calamus scriptorius*, χάλαμος γραφιχός *writing pen*. These two physicians were rivals and founded rival schools. Herophilus was a close follower of Hippocrates. Erasistratus was more independent and explained diseases by mechanical theories, but employed a large number of drugs. His school was followed by the empirics, (Greek ἐμπειριχός, skilled experienced) who believed that all knowledge of medicine was obtained from clinical experience. A rival school, the *methodists* (Greek μεθωδίσται followers of a definite track ὁδός) soon gained the ascendency and the empirics were looked upon as charlatans, so that the word, though honorable in its origin, is still applied to quacks.

We meet with no more epoch marking names until the time of Galen (130–209 A. D.) a physician of the Alexandrian School who stands next to Hippocrates in the ancient medical world. He was an ardent admirer of the older medical writers and an enthusiastic investigator in unexplored regions of medical science. The veins of the brain substance, *venae Galeni*, commemorate his name. Previous to his time, a speculative tendency had crept into all the sciences. Physicians were more interested in elaborating theories of disease, than in applying inductive methods of thought to medical matters. Galen saw that scientific medicine must be based upon a thorough knowledge of anatomy and physiology, that the normal must be known before its abnormal could be explained and corrected. He devoted much time to these elementary branches and made some important discoveries. He demonstrated the existence of the periosteum and described the nutrition of bone; he showed that symphyses were in early life articulations. He discovered that muscles were the organs of locomotion and not mere inert masses for covering bones and viscera; that arteries contained blood and not air as was formerly supposed; and finally he showed the distinction between nerves and tendons.

The rise of Christianity now arrested the development of medical science which came to be looked upon as a black art. Anthropotomy was prohibited and the general belief in dæmoniacal possession, as taught in the New Testament, encouraged the existence of a host of impostors who claimed to cure disease by invoking divine aid. The Cross that brought light to religion, cast a gloom over philosophy and the sciences which soon lulled them to sleep in monasteries or sent them into exile among the Arabians. Thus we find few Greek writers on medicine after Galen who added anything to the science.

Oribasius, court physician to the Pagan Emperor Julian the Apostate, compiled a work of great historical value but evincing little original research, unless we may ascribe to him the discovery of the salivary glands. Soranus wrote the first work on gynaecology and describes the speculum rediscovered in modern times. Alexander of Tralles advanced some new views on pathology, while Paul of Aegina wrote on surgery and obstetrics. We have thus a series of Greek writers on medicine extending from 450 B. C. to 700 A. D. During all this time no discovery of any moment was made by a Latin writer, and even after the decline and fall of Greek learning, the true science of medicine did not pass to the Romans but to the Arabs.

To sum up the influence of Greek science upon the language of medicine we may state that in anatomy the names of the majority of organs requiring careful research for their discovery are taken from the Greek. Thus the names of the external bones of the cranium are Latin, e. g. *frontal, parietal, occipital* and *temporal,* while those requiring dissection for their discovery are Greek, e. g. *ethmoid* and *sphenoid.* From the Greek, also, come the names of nearly all diseases and symptoms. So readily are compounds formed in Greek which express exactly the idea named that scientific men turn instinctively to that language to form the symbols of their thoughts. For this reason we find almost the entire nomenclature of bacteriology to be of Greek origin although the words have nearly all been coined within the past decade. Thus we have:—*Schizomycetes* from σχίζω to split and μύχης fungus; *Micrococcus,* from μικρός small and κόκκος a seed or berry; *Saprophyte,* from σαπρός rotten and φυτόν plant, all being words which designate accurately the thing described. The names of many surgical instruments, such as *lithotrite,* stone pulverizer, from λίθος a stone and τρείβω to pulverize; *cranioclast* a skull crusher, from κράνιον cranium and κλάζω to crush, and of the great majority of operations, e. g. *thoracentesis* boring the thorax from θώραξ the chest and κεντάω to bore, are also mere Greek words in an English dress.

The Latin Element. The student will naturally enquire why the language of medicine is, in structure, Latin, when it is so largely derived from the Greek. Circumstances having no direct bearing upon the development of the science have accomplished this result. The first and only work on pure Roman medicine is from the pen of Cato the Censor, who lived some two hundred years before Christ. It is included in a treatise on rural

affairs, "*De Re Rustica*," and contains about as much
scientific medicine as a similar work composed by "Sit-
ting Bull," or "Tippoo Tib" might be expected to dis-
play. It abounds in superstitious nonsense and slanders
of the regular physicians who were coming to Rome
from Greece about that time. Nevertheless, Cato's work
is significant from a literary point of view. The words
employed by him to express many morbid conditions
and parts of the body were used in the subsequent
translation of Greek works into Latin.

After the fall of Grecian independence, 146 B. C.,
many Greek physicians found their way to Rome. Some
were slaves, others were freemen who came to try their
fortunes. In fact, all the arts and sciences, good and
bad, so highly developed by the Greeks, gained a foot-
hold in Rome, and this sturdy race of warriors was
made effeminate by their captors. As Horace relates, in
his *Ars Poetica:*

> "*Græcia capta ferum victorem cepit, et artes
> Intulit agresti Latio.*"

There was some opposition on the part of the
Roman populace to the new art of medicine, which, to a
certain extent, antagonized their religious notions. Arca-
gathus, the first Greek physician, was dubbed *carnifex,*
meat-maker or butcher, as some surgeons are called by
unappreciative people at the present day, and later
Cato accuses the Greek doctors of having formed a con-
spiracy to poison the Roman nation. But the art of
medicine, thus established on Latin soil, soon took root,
and, for many centuries, maintained a sickly existence
in a Romanized form.

The Roman mind possessed but little originality
except in politics and war. Even the most famous of
the Latin writers were often little more than good trans-

lators. Virgil, in his Eclogues, makes a fair translation of the Idyls of Theocritus, and, in the Æneid, the thoughts, the form, and the poetical figures are, as a rule, taken bodily from Homer.   So in medicine the Romans merely copied from the Greeks.   When a convenient Latin word was wanting, in making their translations, they never stopped to coin one of their own, but took the Greek word and dressed it in Roman type and terminations.   For example, the first section of the small intestine was called in Greek, δωδεκαδάκτυλον, twelve fingers, meaning that this organ was, in length, equal to the width of twelve fingers.   In Latin this was translated *duodenum*, by twelve.   But *ileum*, the name of the third portion of the small intestine, is identical with that used by the Greeks, viz:—*εἰλεόν* or *τὸ ἔντερον εἰλεόν, the twisted gut.* Sometimes the Greek word found its way into Latin, even when there was a good Latin word in existence.   Thus, for liver, there are both the old Latin word, *jecur*, and the Greek, *hepar*, ἧπαρ; for spleen there is the Latin *lien* and the Greek *splenium*, σπλήν; and for amber there is the Latin *succinum*, from *succus*, juice, and the Greek *electrum*, ἤλεκτρον.   The names of diseases and of obscure organs were, almost without exception, borrowed and not translated.

The two most distinguished Latin writers on medicine were Celsus, who flourished from B. C. 53 to 7 A. D., and Pliny the Younger, 23–105 A. D.   Perhaps neither of these men was a physician.   The second speaks in a very deprecatory manner of the art of medicine, but the first displays much practical knowledge. But their works are encyclopædias of the medical knowledge of their time, and Celsus is regarded as the perfection of medical Latinity, even at the present day.   Cœlius Aurelianus wrote on acute and chronic diseases, "*De*

Celeris Passionibus" and *"De Tardis Passionibus."* He
is noted for the purity of his Latin, and his attempt to
avoid, as far as possible, the introduction of pure Greek
words. The monastic physicians, a few years later, read
his work to the exclusion of all others, and, in this
manner, his influence upon the subsequent medical Latin
was very great.

Celsus, Pliny and Aurelian are the only important
Latin medical authors of the classical period. They were
much read by the Latin writers who lived after the
revival of learning, and thus have had a lasting influence
upon our language, if not upon our methods of practice.

When the Roman Empire fell, it dropped into the
lap of the Church, which straightway proceeded to
despoil it of its system of government, thus becoming, for
many centuries, the greatest of temporal powers. The
old pagan literature and philosophy were locked up in
cloisters or destroyed by papal command. The arts and
sciences, with the exception of war, theology and law,
were, to a great extent, suppressed. The scientific medical works composed by heathen writers, and filled with
allusions to strange gods, were among the first to disappear, and physicians who showed any familiarity with
them were regarded as being in league with the evil one.

But the monks began to cultivate, in a rude way,
the arts and sciences. Some whiled away their lonely
hours in the perusal of medical works, and often on their
frequent begging expeditions, in a very unscientific manner, they practiced the healing art. Surgery fell into the
hands of barbers, and not until the tenth century, when
the monks of Salerno began to teach medicine, was there
a medical school in Europe outside of Moorish Spain.
In this school at Salerno surgery was again taught, and
there is some evidence that animals were dissected, for

about this time a work was written on the anatomy of the
hog, "*Anatomia Porci.*" In the twelfth century the
Crusades brought the nations of Europe into contact
with Saracenic culture, and medical works were
translated from Arabic into mediæval Latin. Medicine
then became a purely Arabic science, and so continued until, in the latter part of the fifteenth century, the
ancient medical authors were again studied in the original Greek. About this time practical human anatomy
was revived. Achillini, Berenger, Fallopius, Arantius,
Eustachius, and Varolius of Italy, with Sylvius and
Vesalius of France, form a galaxy of anatomical investi-
gators who have given their names to many of their discoveries. Their works were all published in the sixteenth century, and in Latin, the language of the Church
and State in all Western Europe at this time. Their
style was far purer than that of their monkish prede-
cessors, who had corrupted the language of medicine by
the introduction of numerous Arabic and Moorish-Greek
terms, such as *meri* for œsophagus, *sumac* for the
umbilical region, *myrac* for the abdomen, *siphac* for the
peritoneum, *zirbus* for omentum, and *nucha* for cervix.
This word *nucha* is almost the only Arabic-Latin word
still remaining in anatomical nomenclature, as seen in
ligamentum nuchæ, the ligament of the nape of the neck.

In the latter part of the sixteenth century, medical
men in England began to write in their own language,
although the great majority of the text-books in all the
sciences were Latin, and professors in the schools lectured
in that language. The first English work on anatomy
was compiled by John Banister, in 1578, and was entitled,
" The Historie of Man, from the most Approved Anath-
omistes in this Present Age." In other countries of
Europe, Latin was still the only language of the physi-

3

cians, and so continued far into the eighteenth century. Even at the present day, in Italy, Germany, and Spain, monographs are occasionally composed in Latin, although as a literary language it is fast disappearing. In Germany there is now a tendency to abolish Latin and Greek terms and substitute pure German words. Thus we find them using *krebs* for cancer, *kehlkopf* for larynx, *magenentzuendung* for gastritis, *frauenheilkunde* for gynæcology, etc. In the German language this change is possible, though, perhaps, not advisable. In English, however, it would be very difficult to form words to take the place of our scientific technical terms derived from the Classic tongues. "Windpipehead," "womanhealing-art," and "straightgutinflammation," would certainly be no improvement upon the learned words now employed. Moreover, our colloquial vocabulary is in a constant state of change, as will be shown in a future chapter, whereas, scientific truths, once established, should have names to designate them in all times and in all countries. Where there are several common names for the same thing, much confusion would, in a short time, be introduced into the language of medicine, were the Classical terms to be dropped. What one of the hundred vulgar names for the male organ of generation, which Rabelais has taken the trouble to record in French, could we substitute for the Latin *penis?*

Before leaving the discussion of the Latin element in medicine, we must call attention to the fact that many of our technical words belong to Low Latin, and would not be found in the works of Cicero or Celsus. For example, *scorbutus*, scurvy, is derived from the Teutonic *schaar*, torn, and *buuk*, belly, and *embrocatio* from Greek ἐμβρέχειν, to soak in, both being Mediæval Latin. Sometimes we have both the Classical and Mediæval

Latin word for the same thing, as the following illustrations will show:

CLASSICAL LATIN.	MEDIÆVAL LATIN.	ENGLISH.
pila	bulla	ball
anthemis	chamomilla	chamomile
os frontis	glabella	frontal bone
os	bucca	mouth
equus	caballus	horse

Sometimes we have adopted in medicine the later meaning of words instead of the signification found in the classics. Thus *curatio*, from *curo*, to care for, has come to mean cure, just as from the Greek θεραπών, who was originally a slave or menial who waited upon a master, is derived the modern *therapeutist* who is quite a different person. The ancient word for healing was *medicatio* from *medcor* to heal, and a *medicus* was a healer, at first of wounds, afterward of all diseases, just as was the case with the Greek ἰατρός. Our word *heal* has a similar history. It is derived from a root *hel* meaning *cover*, and from it *heal*, *heel* and *hell* are all formed. To *heal* meant originally, to *cover* a wound with skin; the *heel* is *covered* by the leg, and *hell* is a *covered* place somewhere below.

Latin words are still being formed, and it is anything but a dead language. Antimonium, potassium, and tannicum are words unknown to the Ancients. The recently formed Greek words all wear Latin dresses; we do not write γονοκόκκος but *gonococcus*, nor μυριγγῖτις but *myringitis*. Many of the medical words imported from the modern languages are, when it is possible, promptly turned into Latin. Although we do not inflect *tolu* as a Latin word, we form from it the adjective *tolutanus*. Spanish, Portuguese and Italian words, like *cas-*

carilla, ipecacuanha, and *scarlatina,* are usually treated as if they were Latin, forming a genitive in *æ.*

The nomenclature of a recently-developed branch of our science, medical jurisprudence, is almost exclusively Latin. The rudiments of forensic medicine are found in that mine of legal knowledge, the "Institutes of Justinian," where such subjects as prolonged gestation, sterility, impotence and hermaphroditism are discussed. The technical terms employed by the Latin legal writers have passed through Norman French, and into the English codes, from which our laws are so largely derived.

The Arabic Element. While philosophy and the sciences in Christian countries, during the middle ages, were in a state of slumbering decay, the Arabs, imbued with the wisdom of Indians, Egyptians and Greeks, kept the sacred flame of knowledge burning. Their sages made translations of the *Ayur Veda,* the commentaries of Charaka and Susruta, and cultivated the occult sciences of that mysterious race, the Egyptians. Much of their medical knowledge was derived from the works of Hippocrates and Galen, and, as the Arabic language does not possess that capacity for word-building which belongs to the Greek, many Greek words, slightly modified, were adopted into their vocabularies. The Arabs did not permit the dissection of animals or human bodies. In their manuscripts no drawings of any living thing were permitted, and, as a consequence, there could be no discoveries in anatomy, physiology or surgery. But in the departments of chemistry, materia medica, pharmacy and nosography, great advances were made, which have exerted an influence on medical science felt even at the present day.

Chemistry, or rather alchymy, is distinctively a science of Arabic origin. Many have supposed that the Saracens obtained it in a rudimentary state from Egypt, and, to support this view, claim that the word is derived from *Chemi*, the Egyptian word for Ham, who was, according to the Old Testament, the first settler in Africa. This word *Chemi* was converted by the Greeks into *Ammon*, as seen in Ζεὺς Ἄμμων, although this word may also be derived from ἄμμος, sand, Jupiter Ammon thus meaning "Jupiter of the Sands." The majority of philologists, however, claim that *alchymy* is derived from the Arabic *al*, the, and the Greek χυμεία, pouring or mixing, from χέω, to pour, thus shutting off the etymological argument in favor of the Egyptian origin of this science, making the word mean "the mixing science," instead of the Egyptian or Hamitic science.

The alchemists had two objects constantly in view, first, to discover "the philosopher's stone," which would convert the baser metals into gold, and, second, to find the source of life, or compound a mixture which would enable mankind to retain perpetual youth. In order to accomplish this, they sought for a universal solvent, *alkahest*, which would reduce substances to the four primitive elements of which they believed all things composed. This word *alkahest* was sometimes translated *quintessentia*, fifth essence, by the Latin alchemists, and the word still survives in this form, with altered meaning, in nearly all European languages. Many of the works of the alchemists were composed in cipher, in order that the uninitiated might not learn of their discoveries, and it is now quite impossible to translate them. This custom led an old Latin writer to say: "Alchymy is a great science, for few can understand the language thereof." Wild as were their schemes, and obscure as were their methods, great discoveries were, nevertheless, made. They invented the method of preparing the mineral acids, calling nitro-hydrochloric acid the "royal water," *aqua regia*, as translated in Latin, because it would dissolve gold, the royal metal. Brandy also, was, first prepared by them, and, for a long time, was regarded as the elixir of life. *Aqua vitæ*, it was called by the Latin writers, a name which it still retains in France and Italy as *eau de vie* and *acqua vita*. It also had this name among the Spaniards at one time, but is now called *aguardiente*, burning water, being nearly a literal translation of the German *brandy*, *i. e.*, burning.

The classic period of Arabian medicine began with Rhazes of Persia, 920 A. D., who was the first to describe small-pox and measles in an intelligent manner. In fact, it is to him that we owe our first knowledge of the exanthematous diseases.

Messua, who lived in the eleventh century, wrote an extensive treatise on materia medica, which was translated into Latin in the fifteenth century, passing through twenty-six editions, and finally becoming the basis for the formation of the first London Pharmacopœia, in the reign of James I.

Avicenna, "the prince of physicians," was born 980 A. D., and wrote his "*Canon of Medicine*," in the first part of the eleventh century. A hundred years later his work was translated into Latin, and continued to be used as a standard text-book until about 1650. He was the first to mention the use of the obstetric forceps.

Albucasis wrote on surgery and invented the probang. Of the Moors of Spain, Avenzoar and Maimonides the Jew, were the principal authors, and their works were read throughout the civilized world.

The Arabian influence was much greater upon the
art than upon the language of medicine. Arabic, belonging to a family of languages quite distinct from the Indo-
European, could not easily be Latinized. Arabic words
were, therefore, rarely adopted to designate ideas or discoveries, whatever may have been the defects in the
Latin vocabulary. The great majority of the words that
were transferred before the revival of learning were
dropped by the medical writers of the sixteenth century.
We give below a list of the principal Arabic words still
found in medical literature:

WORD.	ARABIC.	SIGNIFICATION.
Alkali	*al* the, *qali* ash	the ashes of glasswort, abounding in soda.
Alcohol	*al* the, *kahal* eye-wash	a fine powder used to paint eyebrows.
Amber	anbar	a rich perfume
Barberry	barbaris	barberry tree
Benzoin	benzoah	a balsam
Borax	buraq	borax
Caraway	carvi	caraway
Carmine	qirmiz	crimson
Cubebs	kubabah	bitter plant
Elixir	*el* the, *iksir* quintessence	the quintessence, phi- losopher's stone.
Myrrh	murr	bitter
Nitre, natron	nitrun	an alkaline earth, from Nitria
Naphtha	naft	bitumen
Sherbet	sharbat	a drink
Sumbul	sumboul	a spike
Syrup	*sharab* drink	sweet wine
Senna	sana	senna
Sumach	summaq	a shrub, sumach

Saffron	za'faran	yellow
Taraxacum	*tarasacon* succory	dandelion
Tartar	*durdig*, dregs	{ because it is obtained from dregs of wine.
Tamarind	tamrhind, *tamr*, palm, and *hind*, Indian	
Zero	sifr through Italian *zefiro*	

As the mediæval translators of the Arabic medical authors were ignorant of philological science, several words derived from non-Arabic sources were introduced into Latin. In these cases the Arabic definite article *al*, or *el*, was, through a mistaken notion, prefixed to words, thus forming hybrids. We have *alembic*, from *al ἄμβιξ*, the cup or vessel for distilling. In some of the older English works we find the word *alembroth* for ammoniated hydrochlorate of mercury. This word is derived from the Arabic *al*, the, and the Chaldaic *embroth*, "the key to knowledge," because the alchemists expected to determine the final composition of matter from this salt. This method of transferring the definite article as a prefix is occasionally observed in words derived from other languages. Thus, the word *alligator* is merely a corruption of *el ligarto*, Spanish for *the lizard*. The English sailors who heard the word knew nothing of Spanish grammar and would naturally speak of *alligartas*, a word found in the language of that erudite scholar, Ben Johnson.

Elements Derived from Other Ancient Languages. The study of the Old Testament and the commercial relations with the East have introduced a few Hebrew and Persian words into the language of medicine.

From the Hebrew we have:—

Cassia, Heb. *qatzah*, to cut, because the bark was cut off.

Cinnamon, Heb. *qinamon*, from *qinch*, a reed.

Manna, Heb. *man hu*, What is this?

Bedlam, a corruption of Bethlehem, where Mary was in child-bed. Afterward applied to the Asylum of St. Mary of Bethlehem.

From the Persian we have:—

Azedarach, from *aza*, a gum, a plant with anthelmintic properties.

Asafœtida, from *aza*, name of gum, and Latin *fœtida*, stinking.

Bezoar, Persian *padzahar*, from *pad*, against, and *zahar*, poison; whence,—

Bezoardics, remedies used for the prevention of disease.

Cinnabar, from Persian *zinjarf*, red lead.

Jasminum, from Persian *yasmin*, jasmine.

Jujube, corrupted from Pers. *zizafun*, the jujube tree.

Julep, from Pers. *gulab*, rose-water, a sweet drink.

Laudanum, Greek λήδανον, from Persian *ladan*, the gum of the herb, *lada*.

Limon, from Pers. *limun*, lemon or lime.

Orange, Latin *aurantium*, from Pers. *naranj*.

Nard and spikenard, Pers. *nard*, an odor.

Elements Derived from the Modern Languages. During the present century, and, especially, since the Napoleonic wars, a large number of foreign words, especially from the French, have found their way into the language of medicine as used by English-speaking authors. Increased facilities for travel, the telegraph, and the host of medical journals, afford remarkable advantages for the interchange of scientific thought. So rapidly are new discoveries heralded throughout the civilized world that we do not stop to translate new terms but adopt, without change, the word coined by the inventor or discoverer.

Thus words from the French, German, Spanish, and even from the far distant countries of the Orient have found a place in our medical literature. When Piorry wrote his work on percussion, and Laennec published his discoveries in auscultation, English writers did not, at first, stop to frame new words for the terms used to designate these discoveries and, as a consequence, we find the nomenclature of physical diagnosis replete with French words. In neurology, obstetrics, and venereal diseases, branches of medicine carefully studied in France, we also have a number of French words. From Germany and the Scandinavian countries we derive the names of some minerals and of a few diseases. From the Spanish and Portuguese we have obtained the names of many plants and of a few pathological conditions. From the Italian, also, a few words are derived, although this language is so much like the Latin that we generally prefer the Latin equivalents.

Commerce has brought words into our language, as well as merchandise into our markets. From Turkey we have coffee, Turkish *qahveh*, Latinized into *caffea*. From Hindoostan we have *shampoo*, Hindoostani *champna* to rub or press. From the Malay Peninsula we have *gutta-percha*, Malay *gatah*, gum, and *percha*, the tree from which it is obtained; *camphor*, Malay *kapur barus*, barous chalk, Latinized into *camphora*; *rum*, Malay *rum booze*, good drink, and *mango*, Malay *mangga*. From China we have *tea*, Chinese *te*, Latinized into *thea*. From Annam we have *gamboge*, derived from the name of the Province Cambodia, where the plant grows. From a common African personal name we have *Quassia. Quashi* was a West Indian slave, and a "medicine man," who first pointed out the uses of this plant. In slavery days the name *Quashi* was frequently met with among our Southern negroes. We have the plantation song:

> " *Quashi* scrapes the fiddle string,
> And Venus plays the flute."

From the Abyssinian we have *kousso* or *kusso* and *kamala*. From the Tartar *koumiss* or *kumyss*. From the Fijian, *kava-kava*, a word meaning intoxication.

From the American Indian languages through the Portuguese, we have *ipecacuanha*, from *ipecaaguen*, "the roadside sick-making plant," *jequirity* or *jeriquity*, and *jaborandi*. From the Indian languages through the Spanish, we have *boldo, coto, guaiac, jalap* from the Province of Xalapa in Mexico, *kino, quebracho, quinine* from *kina*, bark, *tobacco* from the name of the island of Tobago, *tolu*, the name of a place, and *tonga*, or *tonka*.

From this brief history of the sources of our technical terms, we learn that the language of our science, like the science itself, is truly cosmopolitan, all nations and all ages having contributed to our knowledge and our vocabulary.

CHAPTER III.

The Origin of Words.

WORDS are the symbols of ideas, not mere arbitrary signs such as those used by the mathematicians, but mental pictures addressed to the imagination and recalling the exact relations of the thought symbolized. To be sure these pictures are, in many cases, faded, or as Goethe expresses it, like the images on coins they are worn away by long continued use or obscured by the rust of ages.

Mankind instinctively shrink from the use of words of which they have no accurate knowledge. When foreign words, replete with meaning, are forced upon the common people, they often reform or deform them into words with which they are familiar. The Latin word *carbunculus* means "a little live coal," and was applied to a bright sparkling gem. When these brilliants were introduced into Germany, the Teutonic genius, though obliged to accept the Latin name, converted it into *karfunkel*, from *funkeln*, to sparkle. Many other words have been similarly modified. The German *hausenblase*, fish or sturgeon bladder, has been converted into *isinglass*, the Arabic *carui* into *caraway*, and *benzoin* into *benjamin*. The French *dent de lion*, lion's tooth, has become *dandelion; ros marinus*, sea foam, has become *rosemary; salpetra*, rock salt, has become *saltpetre; verd de gris*, Fr., green of gray, *verdigrease; wermuth*, Germ., mind preserver, *wormwood; cingulum*, the girdle, a Latin name for *herpes zoster*, has been converted into *shingles*, and *staphisagria*, from σταφίς, a vine, and άγρια, wild, has become *stavesacre*. The Spanish *dengue*, a kind of fever common in the Southern United States and Mexico, was called by the English, *danggy* fever, and then "*dandy fever*," a name now found in our medical works. We are also reminded, in this connection, of the physician who told an Irish woman that her husband had pneumonia. "You're right he has *no money*," was her reply.

Words that do not speak to the imagination are things without life. The attempt has been made to form such words in chemical nomenclature, the names of the organic series of compounds being distinguished by the vowel in the final syllable, thus, sext*a*ne, sext*e*ne, sext*i*ne, sext*o*ne, sext*u*ne, and the terminations *ate* and *ite*, have no inherent meaning. The word *sepal* used in botany, it is said, has no etymological signification, having been devised by Neckar, but in this case his mind was influenced by the word *petal*, and, perhaps, by the Latin *sepio*, to divide. Bulwer has modeled his language of the "Vrilya," as given in "The Coming Race," largely after the Greek, and Volupuk, "the universal language," contains the majority of the Indo-European roots.

It is quite probable that the earliest words in all primitive languages were formed by *onomatopœia*, that is, the sound expressing the thing by some peculiar adaptation. When we wish a person to stand we instinctively say *st*. This sound is found as the root of words expressing the idea of immobility in all the Indo-European languages; Aryan *sta*, Greek ἵστημι, Latin *stare*, German *standen*, etc. The first cry of the infant on its entrance into this world is *ma-ma*, and, as its lamentations cease when it is applied to its mother's bosom, our imaginative ancestors employed the word *mamma* as the name of the female breast; thus we have the Greek μάμμα, and the Latin *mamma*, etc. This same root, *ma*, is found in the word for mother in all the Indo-European languages; Sansk. *matri*, Greek μή-ηρ, Latin *mater*, French *mere*, German *mutter*, Russian *mate*, Anglo-Saxon, *moder*, Icelandic *modher*, etc.   Animals were named from their peculiar inarticulate sounds.   The Greek word for frog is βάτραχος, from "*batr-r-r-ach*," the sound which he utters.   From the sound made by the *cow* we get the Sansk. *gao*, Germ. *kuh*, Greek βοός, and Latin *bos*. Names of animals that cannot thus be explained are probably of late origin and are derived from other characteristics.   But even when there are such words we find among the people, and especially with children, a tendency to frame onomatopœic synonymes.   The regular Latin word for cat was *felis*, but *cattus*, the first syllable of which is the sound made by the cat when spitting, is found in colloquial Latin.   So we have *chat* (pronounced *sha*) in French, *katze* in German, all being preferred to words derived from other characteristics.

When people are in strange lands they often go back to the primitive method of word-forming in order to make themselves understood.   A story is told of an Englishman who, on dining in China, wished to know the composition of a certain dish.   Pointing to it he said, "Quack? quack?"   The answer received was, "Bow-wow!"

The sounds made by animals were soon applied to other things.   The winds and torrents roared, as well as the lion.   The *Palatine* Hill takes us back to the days when the shepherds watched their bleating (*balatans*) flocks upon its grassy slopes.   The palate, Latin *palatum*, is the *balatans* organ.   The Latin word for tongue, *lingua*, is derived from the licking sound of the tongue. Compare English *lick*, Greek λείχω, German *lechen*, Italian *leccare*.

The language of the passions is largely onomatopœic.   The Greek γελάσμα, Latin *cacchinatio*, German *lachen*, and English *laugh*, will serve to illustrate this point. In a similar manner words were made to express the sounds of bodies colliding or passing through the air, of ringing, breaking, cracking, splashing, and many others.

These sounds, we believe, were the basis of speech, and were learned by the primæval man as the parrot imitates the sounds he hears. But man has a higher faculty than speech, namely, that of reason, and through this he was enabled to remember, compare and express relations. If he had been created without a larynx, he would undoubtedly have found other means than speech, of communicating his thoughts. As Nodier has aptly said, "Man speaks because he thinks."

From the radical words thus formed by onomatopœia, a host of new expressions may be developed by the addition of prefixes and postfixes. It is said that in the German language there are only about 250 roots, and many of these can be traced to earlier forms; yet, from this comparatively small number of original words, a vocabulary 80,000 strong has been elaborated. To illustrate the formation of words from onomatopœic roots, we may take the radical *ach*, which originally denoted pain, like our *ouch!* In Greek we have ἀκή, a point, ἄκανθα, a thorn, ἄχθος, a burden, etc.; Latin *acuo*, to sharpen, *acus*, a needle, *aculeus*, a spur, *acer*, sharp, etc.; and the same root may be traced throughout the Indo-European family of languages, always having this primary signification of pain, but modified by inflections into a thousand different shades of thought. Indeed, these onomatopœic roots seem to be the true protoplasm of speech, and from a single one, a thousand words often so unlike the original that their relation cannot be detected, are developed. Take, for example, the sound of the initial *m* of *mum*, denoting silence.   In Greek alone there are nearly a hundred words containing this radical.   There is μύω, to close, as seen in *myopia*, in which a partial closing of eyelids is a symptom, *mydriasis*, from μυδρίος, a hot iron which caused the eyes to close and the pupils to dilate, *muscles*, which enclose the viscera, *mucus* (μύκος), phlegm, which is enclosed in the body, μύσος, hatred which one conceals in his mind, μύκης, a mushroom which grows in dim, concealed places, and the *mysteries* of a society are the things that are kept "mum."   *Mutus*, dumb, contains the same root, as do, also, the English words muzzle, mummery and mumps.

Words having meanings very different from the original root are often formed.   Thus, from the root καλ, call, we have the Greek κλύω, to hear.   The word "dear" has two meanings, "prized," because you have it, and "expensive," because you want it.   The Latin word *sacrum* and Greek ἅγιον have the meanings of *sacred* to the gods and *accursed* by the gods.   *Os sacrum* means "*the accursed bone*," because it was not offered up in sacrifices, and not "the sacred bone," as usually translated.

Words are also formed by changing their meaning, *neologisms* of meaning, they are sometimes called.   To illustrate this, we may look at the etymology of the words for man, mankind, and woman.   *Man* is derived from an Aryan root, *ma*, meaning to think or measure, as seen in the Sanskrit *manu*, and *Brahmana*, holy man.   *Kind* is from the Saxon *ge-cynd*, nature. *Mankind* is *man nature*.   Woman was, in Anglo-Saxon, *wifman*, wifeman, becoming in Old English, *wimman*, plural *wimmen*, as pronounced to-day.   The origin of *wife* is not known, but probably referred to her reproductive capacity, as in the sound of the modern wom(b)man.   In Greek the word for man, the male, is ἀνήρ, root (*and*), from an Aryan word meaning testicle. Woman γύνη (root *gynæc*), from γευυάω, to bring forth, produce.   Mankind is ἀνθρωπος, ἀνήρ, man, and ὤζ, looking.   The etymology ἄνω, upward, and τρέπω, to turn, indicating that the primitive man worshipped the sun and stars, is probably a pure fancy.   In Latin we have *vir* for man, referring to his strength, *vis*, allied to Greek ἴς, (root *in*) fibre, strength; for woman we have *femina*, from an old word, *feo*, to produce, as seen in *fœtus, fertile, fecund*, and some other terms; for mankind we have *homo*, allied to *humus*, the soil, because man was formed according to the ancient myth from the earth.

We thus see that language is, as Richter truly says, a dictionary of faded metaphors, using the word metaphor in a generic sense and not subdividing it into the specific rhetorical figures, *synecdoche, metonymy, simile*, etc.   In the recently-developed sciences, such as organic chemistry, figurative language is almost entirely wanting, but in medicine, an ancient art, with a history as old as the human race and bearing in its vocabulary the records of a thousand triumphs, struggles and mistakes, there is an abundance of the poetical method of word formation.

In regard to the metaphorical formation of words, we have: —

1.   *The name of a part or symptom applied to the whole, and conversely.*   In *scrofula*, for example, the neck of a child often swells until it resembles that of a pig, hence the name *scrofula* meaning, literally, a little pig.   In many cases of idiocy the motor apparatus is affected and the patient is obliged to walk with a staff or cane; hence we have *imbecile*, from *in bacillum*, upon a staff or cane.   We now use the word *femur* which means the thigh for *os femoris*, the thigh bone.   In the Hindoo

4

word *beriberi*, we have the symptom for the disease. The limbs in this affection become rigid, and the patient feels as though he were shackled, hence the name from *beri*, a fetter.

2. *The name of a quality or characteristic of an object for the name of the whole.* This method of forming new words is exceedingly common. *Aconite* is so named because it grows upon sharp projecting rocks, ἐν ἀκόναις. *Hydrargyrum* is a watery or fluid silver, ὕδωρ water, ἄργυρον silver. *Paraffin* was so called because it had little affinity, *parum affinis*, for any other chemical substance. *Apocynum* was named from the fact that dogs keep away from it, ἀπό away, κύων dog. Calomel is a *beautiful* remedy for *black* bile, καλός beautiful and μέλας black. *Sarcophagi* were originally made of a stone which was supposed to consume the body, σάρξ flesh, φάγω to eat. The *bregma* is that part of a child's head where sweating or moisture is first observed, from βρέχω to moisten. We speak of the *vagus* or wandering nerve, and call the windpipe the trachea because it is rough, τραχεῖα.

3. *The cause for the effect.* In this class of words we have such as *intertrigo*, to rub together, designating the disease caused by such friction; *nausea*, literally ship sickness, from ναῦς, a ship; and we now hear of people having *malaria*, when they mean they have a disease caused by *malaria* or bad air.

4. *The place for the thing.* In this class of words we have copper, *cuprum*, from Cyprus; *colchicum* from Colchis, Κολχίς, in Asia; *magnesia* and *magnets* from Magnesia a district in Thessaly; *chalybeates*, named from the Chalybes (Χάλυβες), who dwelt in Pontus; *coco* from the province Choco in Mexico; rhubarb from *Rha bar-*

barum, so called because it grew on the wild banks of the river *Rha* or *Volga. Charlatan* comes through the French from the Italian *ciarlatano,* an inhabitant of *Cerreto.* The people of this town were notorious for their boastful language, and we find in Italian the verb *cialare,* meaning to brag. Fom *Tarento* we get *tarantula,* a spider whose bite was supposed to cause the dancing mania of the middle ages, the affection being called *tarantism,* for which about the only remedy was a peculiar variety of music which is still known as the *tarantella.*

Clap, the vulgar word for gonorrhœa is derived from the name of a part of Paris, *Le Clapier,* the word meaning literally a rabbit burrow. This quarter contained numerous houses of ill fame and soon the common French word for brothel was *clapise,* hence the name of the disease acquired in such places.

5. *The name of the inventor or discoverer for the name of the thing.* Every student of human anatomy has observed the common practice of naming a newly discovered part of the body from the person first describing it. Thus we have the fissures of *Sylvius, Rolando,* and *Glasser,* the *lobus Spigelii,* the formanina of *Monro* and *Thebesius,* and many other similar expressions. In physics *Voltaism, Galvanism,* and *Faradism* are named after Volta, Galvani and Faraday who first observed these varieties of electrical phenomena. *Nicotine* and *pelletierine* are derived from the names of Nicot and Pelletier. *Davyum* was named after Sir Humphrey Davy, *krameria* after the botanist Kramer, the *guillotine* immortalizes the name of the supposed inventor Dr. Guillotine, and Dr. Condom has a "*monumentum acre perennius*" in the appliance which commemorates his name.

There is also a large number of plants named in
honor of distinguished persons. *Asclepias*, Greek
'.*Ιαχλέπιας*, is the botanic name of the milkweed. *Juglans* butternut, is the nut of Jove, *Jovisglans*. *Valerian*
is named in honor of the Roman Emperor, *cinchona* is
named after the countess of *Chinchon* who is said to
have been cured by the use of this plant. *Asagraca* is
derived from the name of the distinguished botanist, Dr.
Asa Gray.

6. *The name of the thing derived from something resembling it.* This is pure metaphor and is the commonest
way in which words assume new meanings. Coleridge
has compared words to some of the infusoria which
increase by fission, continually splitting themselves up
into new organisms. This method of growth in language
is remarkably exemplified in tongues having but a comparatively small number of words. The Chinese for
example have only 1500 words and yet these have at
least a 100,000 meanings, and if you will turn to the
word *zug* in your German dictionary you will find over
thirty English words given as equivalents. It is not
necessary to make any extended search to illustrate this
method of word formation.* The *vomer* is the ploughshare, the *tibia*, a flute; the *clitoris*, from Greek *κλεῖς*, a
key, is the door tender; the *testes* are *evidences* of virility;
theobroma is the food of the gods, *θεός* god, *βρῶμα* food.
The little tumors which form in the eyelids are hail-

---

* It is a remarkable fact that synonymes for vulgar or obscene things are always
most numerous, a fact which does no great credit to the natural bent of the human
imagination. Thus we find in the Latin medical writers some 200 names for the *anus,
penis* and *vulva*. Among the Latin names for the male organ of generation are :—
Clava, cauda, columna, gladius, penis, pyramis, radix, ramus, trabs, vas, vena,
and *vomer.*

For the external female genitals we find among a hundred others :—*Annulus,
cava, delta, folliculus, fovea, fundus, hiatus, mesa, ostium, porta, sinus, sulcus,
trema* and *vulva.* These *nomina impudica* all illustrate the formation of metaphorical neologisms.

stones, from the Greek χαλάζων, while *pannus* is a *cloth* growing over the eye.

Sometimes these comparisons are expressed in the form of the words, and not implied as in the above cases. The Greek termination *oid*, from εἶδος, an image, and the Latin termination *formis*, form, being employed. This constitutes a figure of speech denominated by the rhetoricians as *simile.* We have *anthropoid*, manlike, *apes*, and *cuneiform*, wedge-like, bones, as illustrations of this method of formation.

Many words in common use have strange and often obscure etymologies. Many of the dictionaries give no derivation of *syphilis*, yet it plainly comes from σῦς, a hog, and φιλέω, to love. In a poem published by the Italian Fracastoro, *Syphilis* was a swine-herd, very appropriately named, for he certainly ought to have been a lover of hogs. But he unfortunately acquired the *morbus Gallicus*, French disease, as the venereal affection was then designated in Italy.* The French called it *mal de Naples*, the Neapolitan disease, and no nation cared to claim it as their own invention, a fact that induced Voltaire to say: "The pox, like the fine arts, owes its origin to no particular race." As it soon became necessary to have a common word to designate the affection, the name of Fracastoro's swine-herd was adopted into nosology by Sauvage, being peculiarly appropriate, for by a slight change in meaning syphilis means a tendency to have scurfy skin like a hog, just as *hæmaphilia*, blood loving, means a tendency to have hemorrhages.

---

* Quotations from the ancient writers are often given to prove that syphilis existed long before the fourteenth century. We find the following passage in the poems of Perseus, who lived 32–62 A. D. :

"*Tentemus fauces: tenero latet ulcus in ore
Putre, quod haud deceat plebeia raderebeta !*"

But this "*putrid ulcer in the swollen throat*" might apply as well to scarlatina anginosa, diphtheria, or noma, as to syphilis.

The French word *enceinte*, now meaning pregnant, is derived from the Latin *incincta*, girded in. The Roman matron wore a girdle of a peculiar pattern to inform people that she was pregnant and her person sacred. At a later period *incincta* was applied to designate pregnancy, although the women went *un*girdled when in that interesting condition.

The word *dexter*, the right hand, takes us back to the infancy of the Aryan race. This ancient people worshipped the sun, *bhog*, and the south was on the right while thus performing their orisons. The Sanskrit word for south was *dekkan*, allied to *dhu*, shining, and the early meaning of dexter was the south or shining hand. As the sun-god kept to the south, things seen in that direction were looked upon as of good omen as were afterward all things seen on the right hand. Things observed on the left, or north, the region of cold and darkness, were looked upon as unlucky, and so great has been the influence of this myth that many a cultivated lady at the present day feels more comfortable if she first sees the new moon over the right shoulder instead of the left. A *sinister* look is still literally a left-handed, that is, an ill-omened look. Moreover, the right hand is the skillful hand, and *dexterity*, right-handedness, is skillfulness. Among the Romans *sinisteritas*, left-handedness, was awkardness.

The common Aryan word for God was *dyaus*, shining, a word found in the genitive of the Greek *Zeus*, Διός and θεός a god, the Latin *deus* and *Ju*piter, that is, *Diu*pater, shining Father, the Italian *Dio* and the French *Dieu*, all meaning our bright Heavenly Father. It is quite possible, moreover, that our God is only a modification of the Sanskrit *bhog*, the rising sun.

The word used for *soul* or *spirit* in various Indo-European languages, is almost uniformly the same as that for *breath*. The Greek πνεῦμα (*pneuma*), meaning a gas or the soul, is derived from πνέω, to breathe, and the New Testament phrase, τὸ πνεῦμα ἅγιον, usually rendered "Holy Ghost," might from an etymological point of view be translated "sacred wind." So the Latin *spiritus* and our *spirit* are derived from *spiro*, to breathe. The ancients, observing that the soul winged an eternal flight with the cessation of respiration, applied a common word to both.

Van Helmont is said to have invented the word *gas*, and yet, whether conscious of the fact or not, he has made it resemble *geist*, the German word for soul.

In *nightmare* we still see the old Norse demi-god, *Mara*, who was said to strangle people in their sleep.

The *risus Sardonicus*, observed in cases of lock-jaw, is derived from the tradition that in Sardinia there grew a plant which, when eaten, caused people to die of laughter or at least to die laughing.

Delirium is derived from the Latin *de*, off, and *lira*, a furrow or track. When a man is *delirious*, he has wandered from his normal mental track. The same poetical figure is observed in the slang phrase, "off his base."

We have given a sufficient number of examples to prove that imagination and poetry have played an important part in the building and remodeling of words. Sometimes when the origin of words is very obscure men have invented fanciful or legendary derivations. Such etymologies are seen when *formica*, an ant, is derived from *ferens micas*, carrying crumbs; *mors*, death, from *amarus* because it is bitter, or from *Mars* because he is the god of war and death. *Cadaver,** a corpse, has been derived by taking the first syllables of the words *ca*ro *da*ta *ver*mibus, flesh given to the worms. Even the scholarly Archbishop Trench seems to favor the derivation of *crypt*, which evidently comes from χρύπτω, to hide, from "crypit," because sinners in doing penance were placed in pits from which their cries were heard. In this case the cart has evidently been placed before the horse, for *cry pit* is but a corruption of *crypt*. We are reminded of the peasant's explanation of the word *Jew:* "They will *jew* you and *jew* you, and that is why they are called Jews."

Antimony, also, has a legend connected with its name. Basil Valentine was an abbot of a scientific turn of mind. He gave antimony to the hogs upon the monastery farm, and found that they thrived upon it, but when he dosed the monks with the same chemical he learned that it acted with well-nigh fatal violence. On this account he named it *antimonium*, not good for monks, from ἀντί, against, and μόναχος, a monk, or more directly from the French *moine*, a monk.

The word *crystal* is derived from the Greek χρύσταλλος through the Latin *crystallum*, which meant, originally, ice. Michaelis in his work entitled, "The Influence of Language on Opinions, and of Opinions on Language," shows how this word brought a ridiculous error in its train. Pliny tells us that crystals are ice which has been frozen so long that it has forever lost its fluidity; and in St. Augustine, one of the Church Fathers, we read:

---

* 1. *Mors* is derived from Aryan root, *mar*, meaning to die ; *cf.* Sansk. *murtis*, body, *ma rasmus*, etc.

2. *Formica* is cognate with the Sanskrit *vamraka*, an ant, from the root *vam*, meaning to vomit. So named because the ant, when held in the hand, discharges *formic* acid. *Formication* is the name of a symptom in which the patient has the sensation of ants crawling over the skin.

3. *Cadaver* is derived from *cado*, to fall, and was first applied to the bodies of those who had fallen in battle. *Cf.* Greek *ptoma*, a corpse, from *pipto*, to fall. From *ptoma*, the word, *ptomaine*, a cadaveric alkaloid, is derived.

"What is a crystal? Snow hardened into ice for so many years that it cannot readily be dissolved by sun or fire."

We still employ the word *gonorrhœa*, from γόνη, semen, and ῥέω, to flow. although we know it is a flow of muco-pus.

As an example of the manner in which ideas influence language we may cite the notion of the alchemists who believed that there was sex in metals. Arsenic is derived from ἀρσενικός masculine, from ἄρσην a male. Silver was feminine and was sacred to Diana or the moon, *Luna*, a myth which has influenced medical practice even down to the present day. Dr. Martin tells us that nitrate of silver, still called *lunar* caustic, was first administered in epilepsy because it was supposed that epileptics were under the malign influence of the moon, as were all *lunatics*. It followed by a natural course of reasoning that the moon's metal, silver, must be the specific for all moon blasted patients, and this remedy continued its popularity until a few years since, the bromides became the fashionable drug in this affection.

Pliny tells that "*sordes hominis, sudor et oleum,*" that is, "the dirty sweat and grease of man," are sovereign remedies for *angina*. As a consequence of this fallacy how many a quinsied youth has had a dirty stocking wound about his neck at night by his anxious but not over-scientific mother.

The nomenclature of the brain, moreover, shows how ideas may influence language. Our anatomical fathers believed that in the encephalon the homologues of all the parts of the body, both male and female, could be found in miniature; and if you will turn to your text book on anatomy to the description of the brain you will find arms *brachia*, legs *crura*, knees *corpora geniculata*, breasts *corpora mammillaria*, five stomachs *ventriculi*, one of which was anciently called the womb, *utriculus*, a *vulva cerebri*, buttocks *nates*, testicles *testes;* a penis, *clava;* a vulgar name for the pubic hair, *flocculus;* a veil, *velum interpositum*, and a marriage bed, *thalamus*. With all this procreative apparatus before us, we are not surprised to find a union *fornix*, and numerous offspring, quadruplets, *corpora quadrigemina*.

CHAPTER IV.

The Life and Death of Words.

IT is a common error to suppose that words, especially
scientific terms, are born, as was Minerva from the
head of Jove, complete, eternal and unchangeable. One
of the advantages claimed for Latin in scientific nomenclature is that, being a "dead" language, the words will
not be subject to those continual alterations observed in
all modern tongues. The language of Homer is quite
different from that of Sophocles who lived five hundred
years later. Piers Plowman and Chaucer are unin-
telligible to the average English student of to-day. Italian
is but a modified Latin, and in the language of medicine
the student would find considerable difficulty in com-
prehending Banister in his "Anathomy of Man."

To be sure, many of our medical terms are identical
with those employed 1800 years ago by Celsus, whose
style has served as a model for medical writers down
almost to the present decade. Jonathan Pareira, in a
work published as late as 1870, advises the student to
read Celsus in the original in order to acquire an elegant
and accurate medical Latin style.

The alterations in the form of medical words may
be traced most readily by studying a few terms which
have found their way into the language of the people and
have thus undergone changes corresponding to those of
their vulgar lay associates.

Horne Looke, in his work entitled "Winged Words,"
has called attention to the fact that words in their progress through the ages, like regiments of soldiers on
the march, are liable to lose letters and syllables as the

latter are liable to lose soldiers by sickness, casualty and desertion. The word *eleemosynary*, from the Greek ἐλεημοσύνη, consisting originally of twelve letters and seven syllables, has become *alms*, in which only four letters and a single syllable remain.

The classical medical word *hemicrania*, from the Greek ἡμικρανία, *half a skull*, became in Low Latin *migræna* by a process of clipping and alteration, just as in the vulgar English of to-day we hear people saying "morphydite" for "hermaphrodite," "janders" for *jaundice*, which is itself a corruption of the French *jaunisse*, yellowness, and "anguintum" for *unguentum hydrargyri*. From this mediæval Latin word *migræna* the French *migraine*, often used in medical works, was formed, and *migraine*, when it traveled across the English Channel, was changed into *megrim*, a word recognized in all our medical dictionaries.

The Greek κυνάγχη, *cyanche*, from κύων, a dog, and ἄγχω, to choke, that is, to choke like a dog, became in Low Latin *esquinantia* from which the French *esquinancie* and our *quinsy* have been formed.

Paralysis, Greek παράλυσις, an abnormal loosening, or loosening on the side, became in middle English, *parlesy*, and in modern English *palsy*. *Hydrops*, Greek ὕδρωψ, a watery appearance, became *hydropisie* in Old French, *ydropsie* in Old English, and *dropsy* in the modern vernacular.

Rachitis, Greek ῥαχῖτις, an inflammation of the spinal column, has become *rickets* in the vernacular, although it has been claimed that *rachitis* is derived from *rickets* and that *rickets* is derived from the Anglo-Saxon *wringan*, to twist. *Cataract*, as applied to opacity of the crystalline lens, is commonly derived from καταρράκτης, a rushing down, a word which is not at all suited to the nature of the disease. The word was probably *catarapt*, from the Greek καταῤῥάπτης, a covering over, the crystalline lens having the appearance of being covered over with a white film or cloth. But as people could see no real meaning in *catarapt* it was changed, according to the law mentioned in the preceding chapter, into *cataract*, a word with which they were already familiar.

Glycyrrhiza, from the Greek γλυκύῤῥιζα, sweet root, was early corrupted into the Latin *liquiritia*, and in English into liquorice and licorice. Trench, however, inclines to the belief that liquorice is derived from *liquor* as Fuller uses the expression "glycyrrhize or liquoris." But this may have been due to Fuller's ignorance of the origin of the word. Tansy comes to us through the Latin *tanacetum*, which, in its turn, is a corruption of *athanasia* (ἀθανασία) immortality.

Many Latin words used in medicine have undergone similar changes. *Inula campana* has become *elecampane: lactucarum, lettuce; bipennula, pimpinella;* and *barbascum* is now known as *verbascum*. *Eglantine* is only a modification of *aculentinus*, and the Spanish *cebadilla*, a diminutive of *cebada*, barley, is now found in our works on materia medica as *sabbadilla*.

We have only to glance at the last American Pharmacopœia to convince ourselves that changes are continually taking place in the language of medicine. The gender of the Latin terms for the salts ending in *as* and *is* was changed in 1880 from feminine to masculine. From 1860–1880, *calcii carbonas precipitata* was the proper officinal name for precipitated chalk; now it is written *calcii carbonas precipitatus*. The names of all the alkaloids previously ending in *ia*, such as *morphia, strychnia* and *quinia*, were modified so that the ending is now *ina*; thus, *morphina, strychnina* and *quinina*. The

names of neutral principles had their terminations changed
from *ina* to *inum*, being made neuter instead of feminine.
Sulphuretum was changed to *sulphidum*. *Arsenicum,
manganesium, brominium, iodinium* and *chlorinium* were
contracted into *arsenium, manganum, bromum, iodum*
and *chlorum*. *Chiretta* was changed to *chirata, assafœtida*
to *asafœtida, gambogia* to *cambogia, glycerina* to *glyceri-
num*, and *pyroxylon* became *pyroxylinum*.

Adjectives derived from words thus changed were
also remodeled; thus, *chlorinatus* became *chloratus*, and
arseniatus, arsenatus. *Redactum* was supplanted by
reductum. The gender of *rhus* was changed from neuter
to feminine. Similar changes have been made in the
nomenclature of diseases, and in other departments of
medical science.

Your attention has already been called to the fact
that words, like the cells of animals, die when their
natural functions have been fulfilled. In Greek the older
word for gold (αὖμος) was early dropped for χρυσός, the
necessary, and thousands of words in the older English
works are never heard in conversation to-day. During
the last half century there has been a great decline in the
use of Latin in medicine. Only fifteen years ago Dr.
Pereira mentions in one of his works that he knew an
eminent hospital surgeon who confessed his inability to
write directions to the patient in his prescriptions in correct Latin, while at present it would be quite as remarkable to discover a surgeon who could truthfully admit
the contrary. A host of terms connected with blood-
letting have disappeared from our medical works. Such
words as *melanagogue, acopa, antiloimica, antiscolica,
bezoardic, phtheiroctonia* and *alæphangina* seem strange
to the modern practitioner. Directions to the patient
are, in America, no longer written in Latin, for our drug-

gists could not translate them. Even the common expression, "*pro re nata*" has been rendered "for the baby just born." "*Maneat in lecto*," "let the patient remain in bed," has been translated, "to be taken in milk in the morning," while "*mane in lacte*" has been rendered "remain in bed."

But a few years have elapsed since the pharmacopœias of various nations and colleges were uniformly printed in Latin. The first United States Pharmacopœia was printed in both Latin and English. The modern Greek Pharmacopœia is printed both in Latin and the vernacular, but with this exception, Latin has been quite generally abandoned except in nomenclature.

Moreover, old remedies and names for diseases are constantly disappearing. *Lyssa* gave way to *hydrophobia*, and this is now very properly being abandoned for *rabies*. The once popular remedy, a *pilula perpetua*, a pill made of metallic antimony, which had perpetual virtues of a cathartic nature, and could be used by any number of patients, is no longer employed, and we hear as little now of *arteriotomy*, first practiced by Aratæus, as we do of Bishop Berkeley's tar water cure or of " Perkins' tractors."

Turning again to the last edition of the U. S. Pharmacopœia, we observe that although the names of many remedies have been changed, at least as many more have been dropped in ten years. We do not mean to say that the board of scientific gentlemen who have charge of the revision of the Pharmacopœia once in ten years are endowed with verbicidal powers, yet they give stunning blows to many words which at first cause them to fall into disuse and then into decay. After the lapse of a few decades, such words will be brought to light only by the aid of historical research, being lifeless objects, mere skeletons which remind us of a past vitality. It is on account of these numerous mummy words that the student finds so much difficulty in understanding the works of the ancient and mediæval medical authors.

Sometimes the old words remain with altered meaning. *Metria* no longer means womb disease, but puerperal fever, and *hysteria* has far more to do with the nervous system than with the female reproductive organs. *Aristolochia*, from ἄριστος, best, and λοχεία, child-bed, was formerly applied to an entire class of oxytocic remedies, but is now limited to the name of a single plant, *birthwort*, or Virginia snake root.

Still more frequently words become old and decrepit, losing the vigor with which they were once so pregnant. We meet with such archaic expressions in the language of the aged. *Syncope* is now preferred to *deliquium animi*, *intussusception* to *ileus*, and so on.

We thus see that the component parts of a language are in a constant state of change, coming into existence, changing their form, and dying of old age, like beings endowed with life.

PART II.

THE LATIN ELEMENT IN THE LANGUAGE OF MEDICINE.

CHAPTER I.

ORTHOGRAPHY.

THE letters employed in medical Latin are the same in number, power and character as those used in modern English. In classical Latin there was no *j*, *v*, *u* or *w*, while *k*, *x* and *z* were used only in words derived from the Greek. In writing Roman numerals the final *i* was written *j*, thus *viij*, a custom still practiced in writing prescriptions. In the fifteenth century this final *j* was employed instead of *i* to indicate the consonant sound of *y*, and we now ascribe to *j* a sound indicated by *dzh*.

V also is of recent origin and is used to indicate the consonant sound of *u*; and *w*, i. e. *uu*, is merely a new symbol to indicate another consonant sound of *u* before a vowel, as in *equus*, now pronounced *ekwus*. *W* is found in several medical Latin words derived from proper names, *e. g. Corpora Wolfiana, Ossa Wormiana, Waltheria, Wintera* and *Wrightia*. In classical Latin *k* was found only before *a*, but in medical Latin it is found in other positions, for example before *r* in *Krameria*, a word derived from the name of the celebrated Dr. Kramer.

Initial *x*, *y* and *z* are found only in Latin words of foreign origin, thus: *xeroderma*, from ξερός dry, and δέρμα skin; *Yttrium* from *Ytterby*, a Swedish town, and *zymosis*, from ζυμέω, to ferment.

5

The letter *y* was borrowed by the Romans from the Greek to designate the sound of the Greek *upsilon* which differed from the Latin *u*.

The letters are divided into classes as follows: —

1. Vowels: *a, e, i, o, u, y.*

2. Consonants
    - liquids, *l, m, n, r.*
    - mutes
        - labials, *p, b, f, ph* and *v.*
        - palatals, *c, ch g, k, q* and *j.*
        - linguals, *t, th* and *d.*
    - sibilant, *s.*
    - aspirate, *h.*
    - double consonants, *x* and *z.*

X is equivalent to *cs, ks, gs, or chs.*

Z is equivalent to *ds* or *ts.*

CHAPTER II.

ORTHOEPY.

ORTHOEPY is the art of pronouncing words correctly. The ancient pronunciation of Latin has to a great extent been lost and it is extremely doubtful if it can ever be recovered. Numerous attempts have been made to discover and restore the classical pronunciation but all such efforts are based upon hypotheses incapable of demonstration. The English method* of pronouncing Latin should be learned by every student contemplating the study of medicine.

1. Because many Latin words used in medical literature have become thoroughly Anglicised and the use of any other than the English method of pronunciation would sound pedantic, affected, and ridiculous. Such familiar words as *vapor*, *cicatrix* and *vagina* would scarcely be recognized if pronounced *wah' por*, *kee kah'-treex* and *wah ghee'nah*. according to the so-called Continental method.

2. Other Latin words have long been pronounced by the medical profession strictly in accordance with English methods, and the introduction of any other system would only serve to introduce fresh confusion

---

* The literary schools and colleges of this country are about equally divided between the three pronunciations of Latin, *English, Continental* and *Roman*. A small majority of the schools, however, in 1885, still adhered to the English method, while not one educated man in ten would pronounce Latin in accordance with the rules of the Continental or Roman methods. Allen and Greenough, in their Latin grammar, direct the student to pronounce familiar Latin phrases in accordance with the English method, although they advocate the Continental method for use in schools.

Furthermore, every European nation pronounces Latin according to the sounds of the letters in its own language. Why, then, should the English make themselves ridiculous by pretending to restore the ancient pronunciation of the Roman tongue?

A few physicians, displaying more pedantry than good sense, propose to give the Continental sounds of the vowels and retain the English sounds of the consonants in pronouncing Latin medical terms! This method (?) of pronunciation is beneath criticism. Medical technical terms should be regarded as English words borrowed, for convenience sake, from the classical languages.

into medical orthoepy. Not one medical man in a thousand would pronounce *biceps* bee'kapes, or *cilium* ke'le oom.

3. A study of the rules of pronunciation, as applied according to the English method, will be of material assistance to the student in determining the pronunciation of all words found in his text-books, whether they be of Latin or other origin.

For these reasons we advocate the use of the English method of pronunciation of all words used in medical works with the exception of those recently transferred to our vocabulary from the modern foreign languages, such as the French, German and Italian.

In order to pronounce correctly in accordance to the rules of the English method a knowledge of the following particulars is requisite:—

1. Of the *sounds of the letters* in all their combinations.

2. Of the *quantity* of the penultimate syllables of words.

3. Of the *place of the accent*, both primary and secondary.

4. Of the *mode of dividing words into syllables.*

SECTION I.—THE SOUNDS OF THE LETTERS.

I. Of the Vowels:

RULE I.   *A vowel at the end of an accented syllable has its long English sound.*   Examples: Mā'nia, vē'na, vi'num, ō'ra and tū'ba, in which the accented vowels are pronounced as in Jane, mete, wine, go and cube.

Remark. This rule is often violated, in fact usually violated, in the names of inflammatory diseases ending in *itis.* Bronchī'tis is the correct pronunciation, not bronche'tis. You should certainly have a uniform system of pronunciation, and if you use bronche'tis you should also use ki'koom for *cæcum.*

A at the end of an unaccented syllable has the sound of a in father; thus co′cā, mistu′rā.

E, *o* and *u* at the end of unaccented syllables have about the same sound as when accented, but shorter and less distinct; thus re′te, potas′sa, ge′nu.

I final, always has its long English sound; thus mus′culī, au′rī.

I at the end of an unaccented syllable, not final, has its short sound as in *if*, ex. tib′ia.

Except at the end of the first syllable of a word, the second of which is accented, when the long sound is the rule; thus vitel′lus, sī ăl′′a gŏ′gā.

Y is pronounced like *i* in the same situations.

RULE II. *A vowel has its short English sound when followed by a consonant in the same syllable*, e. g. căs′sia, mĕn tā′lis, vīs cŭs, vŏm′ica, bŭlla, in which the vowels are pronounced as in c*a*t, m*e*t, v*i*m, f*o*x, and b*u*t.

Exceptions. 1. *A*, before *r* and a consonant, is pronounced as in English; thus *pars*, as in *part*.

2. *Es* final is pronounced like *ease*; thus pubes.

3. *Os* at the end of plural cases is pronounced like *ose* in *dose*; thus ocul*os*, equ*os*.

II. *Of the Diphthongs :*

1. *Ae* and *oe* are always diphthongs unless separated by a diaeresis. They are pronounced as *e* would be in the same situations; thus *næ′vus* (nē′vus), *hæmatox′ylon* (hĕm′′atox′ylon), *fœniculum* (fēnic′ulum).

2. *Ai, ei, oi* and *yi* usually have the vowels pronounced separately; thus mā′ys, dīē′ī, cō′itus.

3. *Au* when a diphthong is pronounced like *aw* in *saw;* thus, *aura* (aw′rah), *haustus* (haws′tus).

4. *Eu* when a diphthong is pronounced like long *u* ; thus, eūcalyp′tus, eūthana′sia.

Observation. *Eu* at the termination of Latin nouns and adjectives are pronounced separately; thus, nu′cle us, au′re us.

5. *Ua, ue, ui, uo* and *uu* are pronounced like *wa, we,* etc.; thus, *aqua* (ā′kwah), *quercus* (kwer′cus), *liquor* (lī′kwor), *equus* (ē′kwus). They are always diphthongs after *q* and *g*, and sometimes after *s*.

III. Of the Consonants.

The consonants in Latin are usually pronounced like the corresponding English letters in the same situations. Particular attention, however, should be paid to the following rules and cases :

RULE I.   *C has the sound of s and g the sound of j, before e, i and y and the diphthongs æ and œ;* thus, çerium, çicu′ta, çydo′nium, çæ′sium, çœli′aca, gena, gingi′va, gyrus, Gæta.

Observation 1.   It is reasonably certain that *c* and *g* were always hard in the language of the ancient Romans, and furthermore, it is probable that *g* had a sound quite as much like *k* or *c* hard as the sound which we now ascribe to it.

Observation 2.   A few medical scholars are in the habit of giving the hard sound of *c* and *g* before *e* and *y* in words of Greek origin, on the ground that we should assign to these letters the same sounds found in the original language; thus, *gynæcology, cyanogen* and *hyoscyamus* are pronounced ghīne col′ogy, kyanoghen and hyosky′a mus.   But this method of pronunciation is inconsistent with general usage and incorrect, for upon this principle *geometry, genesis,* and *cylinder* should be pronounced gheometry, ghenesis, and kylinder.

RULE II.   *C and g before consonants, the vowels a, o, and u, and diphthongs with the exception of æ and œ, have their hard sounds, i. e., c* has the sound of *k,* and *g* the sound of *g* in *gay;* thus, *cadmium, corium, galbanum, guaiacum,* etc.

Remark 1.   *C* following or ending an accented syllable before *i* followed by a vowel has the sound of *sh*; thus, *acacia* (akashea).

Remark 2.   *G* before *g* soft is assimilated to it in sound; thus, *agger* (ajjer).

Remark 3.   *C* hard before *c* soft is not thus assimilated.   We frequently hear *micrococci* pronounced. by those ignorant of this rule, as if it were spelled microcossi or microcokki.

RULE III.   *Ch* in all pure Latin words and in words of Greek origin has the sound of *k*; thus, *charta, chalazion,* pronounced kär′tah, kälä′zion.

Observation.   This rule is frequently violated.   We often hear *chian* pronounced tchian, *catechu,* catichew, and *colchicum* has been so generally mispronounced that any attempt to restore its proper sound would be vain. The word should be köl'kĭkum, not koltch'ikum, as we usually hear it, although the latter is more euphonious.

Chiretta, or *chirata* according to the revised Pharmacopœia, is an exception to the above rule because the word is not properly Latin but Hindustani, in which language it is pronounced as if spelled tchira'ta.

RULE IV.   *Cm, cn, ct, gm, gn, mn, tm, ps, phth, and pt, at the beginning of words are pronounced with the first letter silent;* thus, *cnicus* (nĭ'kus), *gmelin* (melin), *gnome* (nome), *mnemonics* (nemonics), *tmesis* (mesis), *psora* (sora), *pterygoid* (terygoid), *phtheiri'asis* (thiri'asis).

RULE V.   *S* has usually its hissing sound, as in *so*, *e. g.*, *somnus.*

Exception 1.   *Si* followed by a vowel and immediately succeeded by a consonant in an accented syllable, has the sound of *sh* in *she;* thus, *xanthopsia* (zanthop'shea).

Exception 2.   *Si* followed by a vowel and immediately preceded by an accented vowel, has the sound of *zhe ;* thus, *aphasia* (apha'zhea).

Exception 3.   *S* final, after *e, æ, au, b, m, n* and *r* has the sound of *z*; thus, *res* (rez), *trabs, lens.*   *S* also has the sound of *z* in *rosa, causa* and *residuum.*

RULE VI.   *T following or ending an accented syllable before i followed by a vowel has the sound of sh ;* thus, *fortius* (for'sheus), *Arantius* (aran'sheus).

Exception.   After *s, t* or *x*, in the above situation, *t* retains its hard sound; thus, *pæderastia, sextius.*

RULE VII.   *X* at the beginning of words has the sound of *z*; thus, *Xylophyllum* (zylophyl'lum), *Xanthina* (zanthī'na). *X* at the end of syllables has the sound of *ks*; thus, *axis* (ak'sis).

Exception 1.   When *ex* or *ux* are followed by a vowel in an accented syllable, the *x* has the sound of *gz*; thus, *exemplum* (egzem'plum).

Exception 2.   *X* ending an accented syllable before *i* followed by a vowel has the sound of *ksh*; thus, *noxius* (nok'sheus).

SECTION II.—OF THE QUANTITIES OF THE SYLLABLES.

The *quantity* of a syllable is the relative time occupied in pronouncing it.   But little attention is paid to quantity in the pronunciation of Latin prose. It is necessary, however, to know the length of the penultimate (next to the last) syllable in order to place the accent correctly.

The sign of the long syllable is ($-$), of the short syllable ($\smile$), and of a common syllable, *i. e.* one that is sometimes long and sometimes short ($\asymp$). The student should disabuse his mind of the idea that quantity has anything to do with the sounds of the vowels. For example, *liquor* in Latin has the quantity of the *i* short, but is pronounced lī′quor. *Spiritus* has the first *i* long in quantity, but is pronounced spiritus. This same remark will apply to Latinized Greek words.

The last syllable of a word is called the *ultimate*, the next to the last the *penult*, and the third from the last the *antepenult*.

RULE I. *All the diphthongs except those beginning with u are long.*

RULE II. *A vowel before a double consonant (x, z or j), or before any two consonants, except a mute followed by a liquid, is always long, although it has the short English sound;* thus, ēxtrāc′tūm, metāl′lum, pyrēx′ia, but short in cer′ēbrum, Per′icles.

RULE III. *A vowel before another vowel or diphthong, or before h followed by a vowel or diphthong, is short by nature;* thus, al′līum, ret′rāhens.

Exception. There are numerous words of Greek origin used in medical works in which a single vowel represents a diphthong or the long vowels ω, or η; thus, we have asthenī′a, from ἀσθενεία where *i* is equivalent to the Greek ει; achillē′a, from the Greek ἀχίλλεια, and hydrozō′a, from ὑδροζῷα. In these cases the vowel representing the diphthong or long letter is always long in quantity regardless of position.

In other cases, where the above rules are not applicable, it is necessary to learn the quantity of the penultimate syllable. The student, for example, must know the *i* in the termination *ina* applied to the names of alkaloids in long; thus, quinī′na, morphī′na; but the *i* is the termination *idum* in short; thus brom′idum, iod′idum. *A* in the termination *as* is long; thus phosphā′tis, nitrā′tis, etc.

SECTION III.—OF THE ACCENT.

RULE I. *In words of two syllables the penult is always accented.* Examples, fē'mur, ul'na. rā'phe.

RULE II. *In words of more than two syllables, if the penult is long in quantity it is accented, but if short, the accent is on the antepenult.* Examples, acē'tum, hydrăs'tis, orchi'tis, ac'ĭdum, ce'rium, an'thĕmis.

Words of more than three syllables may have two accents, a primary and a secondary, as *hy''drocyan'idum.* The rules for determining the place of the secondary accent are as follows :

RULE III. *If only two syllables precede the primary accent, the secondary accent is placed upon the first syllable;* Examples, *hae''matox'ylon, pros''tat'i'tis.*

RULE IV. *When more than two syllables precede the primary accent, the secondary accent is placed sometimes on the first and sometimes on the second syllables.* Examples, *per''itoni'tis, ventric''ulo'rum.*

SECTION IV.—DIVISION OF WORDS INTO SYLLABLES.

Every Latin word is divided into as many syllables as there are separate vowels and diphthongs, thus differing from the English in which there are numerous silent vowels. Examples, rē'tē, Pom pē'i i.

1. *H* between two vowels is joined to the vowel following it, as *tra here.*

Ch, ph, and *th* are treated like single letters equivalent to the Greek, χ, φ, and θ.

2. *Gl, tl,* and *thl,* when standing alone between two vowels, are always separated unless the first vowel be *u.* Examples, *neurog'lia, at'las, ath let'icus.*

3. *X* between two vowels, is united to the vowel preceding it, but in pronunciation its elementary sounds are separated; thus *ax il'la* pronounced ak-zil'la.

4. A single consonant or a mute followed by *l* or *r* between the last two vowels of a word or between the vowels of any two *unaccented* syllables must be joined to the latter vowel; thus *ae ther, ru ber.*

5. A single consonant or mute with *l* or *r* after the vowel of an accented syllable, whether that accent be primary or secondary, is joined to the accented vowel; thus *funic'ulus, helleb'orus, lig''amen'tum.*

6. Two consonants between two vowels must be separated; thus *cor'pus, aph'tha.*

7. When three consonants are placed between two vowels, the last, or if that be *l* or *r* preceded by a mute, the last two are joined to the latter vowel; thus *trans versa'lis, fenes'tra, em plas'trum.*

8. In dividing compound words into syllables, the component parts are to be separated, if the first part ends in a consonant. But if the first part ends in a vowel or has dropped its termination, it is to be divided like a simple word. Examples, ambi dex'ter, semper'virens.

ILLUSTRATIVE EXERCISES IN PRONUNCIATION.

In the following sentences the signs — and ‿ indicate the English sounds of the vowels:

In fīg'ĭ mŭs prāē ter'ĕ ā cū cŭr'bī tăs lĕ'vēs, quāē Grāē cī cū'phăs vō cănt, scĭl'ī cet sī'nĕ scăr'''ī fī cā''tī ō'nĕ. A rĕn'tēs ĕt sĭc'căs cū cŭr bĭt'ū lăs dī'cĭt, quāē ăd mō vĕn'tŭr cŭm flăm'mä. In tĕr'dŭm ĕ'nĭm cŭm ā'quä cál'ī dä áp pŏn''e bā'tur, quĕm ăd'mo dŭm scrĭp'sĭt Al bū cā'sĭs, ca pĭt'ŭlo, "Dē ū'sō cu'cŭr bĭt''ū lā'rŭm. *CAE'LIUS AURELIA'NUS.*

Dē ĭn'dē ĭn ĭp'sä ăr tē'rĭa vē nō'sä, ĭn spĭ rā'tō ā'ĕ rī mĭs cē'tŭr et ĕx spī rā''tĭ ō'nĕ ā fū līg'ī nĕ ĕx pŭr gā'tŭr; ăt'que ī'tem tăn'dĕm ā sĭn ĭs'trō cŏr'dĭs vĕn trĭc'ū lō tō'tŭm mĭxtŭm pĕr dĭ ăs'tō lĕn ăt trā'hĭ tŭr, áp'tä sū pĕl'lex, ŭt fī'ăt spĭr'ī tŭs vī tā'lĭs. Quŏd ī'tä pĕr pŭl mō'nēs fī'ăt cŏm mū'nī cā'tĭ ō ĕt prāĕp ā rā'tĭ ō, dō'cĕt cŏn jŭnc'tĭ ō vā'rī ä et cŏm mū nĭ cā'tĭ o vē'naē ăr tĕr'ī ō'saē cŭm ăr tĕr'ī ä vē nō'sä ĭn pŭl mŏn'ĭ bŭs. Cŏn fĭr'măt hŏc măg nĭ tū'dō ĭn sĭg'nĭs vē'naē ăr tĕr''ī ō'saē, quāē nĕc tā'lĭs nĕc tăn'tä ĕs'sĕt făc'tä, nĕc tăn'tăm ā cŏr'dĕ ĭp'sō vĭm pū rĭs'sī mī săn'guĭ nĭs ĭn pŭl mō'nēs ē mĭt'tĕ rĕt, ŏb sō'lŭm ē ō'rŭm nū trī mĕn'tŭm; nĕc cŏr pŭl mŏn'ī bŭs hăc rā tĭ ō'ne sĕr vī'rĕt, cŭm prāē sĕr'tĭm án'te ä ĭn ĕm bry ō'ne sō le'rĕnt pŭl mō'nēs ĭp'sī ăl''ī ŭn'dē nūtrī'rī, ŏb mĕm brăn'ū lăs ĭl lăs seū văl'vū lăs cŏr'dĭs ūs'quē ăd hō'rŭm nā tĭv ĭ tā'tem; ŭt dō'cĕt Gā lē'nus, etc.

SERVE'TUS.

CHAPTER III.

Words Commonly Mispronounced.

NO class of professional men mispronounce the technical words of their calling more commonly than physicians. This is sometimes due to defective elementary education, but more frequently it results from the blunders and bad example of medical orators and college professors, who, under the influence of the American spirit of freedom, declare themselves independent of all orthoepical and etymological rules. There is, however, but little excuse for these errors so commonly committed by men who place themselves before the profession as teachers, whether it be in the class-room or the medical society. Almost without exception our technical words are pronounced strictly in accordance with well established rules, but these rules are violated occasionally even by the makers of medical dictionaries. Thomas, for example, the most accurate of the medical lexicographers, pronounces *neurog'lia, neurogli'a.* Dunglison commits frequent errors, pronouncing *anæm'ic, anæ'mic,* thus violating one of the primary rules of English orthoepy; * and in a small "pronouncing medical lexicon" a

---

* Many people have the erroneous idea that the pronunciation of English words is a purely arbitrary matter, being determined by common usage and not depending upon any fixed rules. In words derived from the Latin, both the accent and the sounds of the vowels and diphthongs are determined by the English pronunciation of the Latin word. The Latin for *anæmic* is *anæmicus,* which must be pronounced *a nem'icus.* Cutting off the termination *us,* we have *a nem' ic,* the proper English pronunciation.

In polysyllabic words of Latin origin, the place of the accent is determined in a different manner, the secondary accent of Latin words having the primary accent on the penult becoming the primary accent in English. For example, *vag' ina'lis* becomes *vag'i nal,* not *va gi'nal; cer' e bra'lis* becomes *cer'e bral,* not *cer e'bral.*

We cannot, however, entirely ignore the influence of custom in the pronunciation of words. The Latin word *ver ti'go* is almost universally pronounced *ver'-tigo* in English, and common usage has made this pronunciation correct, although it was, at first, an error due to ignorance of the quantity of the penult. These occasional exceptions to the established rules of orthoepy do not prove that pronunciation is a purely arbitrary matter any more than the birth of an occasional monstrosity in the animal world would prove that species are not reproduced in accordance with fixed natural laws.

cursory examination has detected no less than forty of
the most palpable errors.

In order to illustrate the frequency with which words
are mispronounced, we will make use of an excellent
method adopted by Dr. L. P. Meredith in his little book
on "*Errors of Speech.*"

The study of orthoepy was so highly developed
among the ancient Greeks that the mispronunciation of a
single word by an orator was greeted by jeers and hisses.
Let us imagine Prof. Blowmuch, of the X. Y. Z. Medical
College, addressing the ancient class of Dr. Hippocrates:

"GENTLEMEN : — The subject of our dis'course (*hisses*)
to-day will be vario'la (*hisses*), rubeo'la (*hisses*) and varioloid'
(*hisses*). The ètiol'ogy (*hisses*) of these affections is not well
known. Some regard micrococ*k*i (*hisses*) as the *primum*
(*hisses*) *causa*, others seek for fomi'tes (*hisses*). It is quite
certain, however, that the det'ritus (*hisses*) of the pustules
and the fē'tid (*hisses*) odor of the disease contain an infectious
principle. When occurring in ad'ults (*hisses*) each vario'lous
(*hisses*) pustule leaves a cic'atrix (*hisses*) especially in the
fàc'ial (*hisses*) tissues, but the ab'domen (*hisses*) of a patient
with much adipoze (*hisses*) tissue may escape. With regard
to treatment, use àmmo'nìi (*hisses*) aç'etas (*hisses*) for a res'-
piratory (*hisses*) stimulant when ràls (*hisses*) and broo'ys (*hisses*)
are heard in the lungs. Car'minatives (*hisses*) are sometimes
indicated. Correct constipation with podoph'yllum (*hisses*)
and hyoscyà'mus (*hisses*), removing s*k*ybalæ (*hisses*) by means
of an ene'ma (*hisses*). For local antisepsis, I prefer iò'doform
(*hisses*) and weak solutions of hydrarg'yrum (*hisses*), chlorī'dum
(*hisses*) corro'sivum (*hisses*). When there is much asthe'-
nia (*hisses*), a suppository of digitàl'is (*hisses*) and co'nium
(*hisses*) may be inserted in àn'o (*hisses*). When death occurs
the clothing and even the cadàv'er (*hisses*) should be sent to
the crē'matory (*hisses*)," etc.

Such blunders as the above are of daily occurrence; in fact the majority of the words in the following list were collected at medical meetings and in the class-room.

Although this chapter is, for convenience sake, placed under the head of the Latin element in the language of medicine, many words not derived from that source have been inserted.

The following are the signs indicating the pronunciation:

ā, ē, ī, ō, ū, as in *ale, mete, kite, dote* and *cube.*
ă, ĕ, ĭ, ŏ, ŭ, as in *mat, bet, bit, bot* and *but.*
ä as in *father.*
ŏŏ as in *govn.*
ōō as in *fool.*
c as in *cat.*
ç as in *cider.*
ch as in *chapter.*
g as in *gad.*
s as in *hiss.*

A.

abdomen, ăb dō'men, *not* ab'do men.
abducens, ăb dū'senz, *not* ab'doo sens.
aberrans, ăb ār'ranz, *not* ab'er rans.
abluens, ăb'lū enz, *not* ab lōō'ens.
abomasus, ăb o mā'sus, *not* ā bŭm'a sus.
acacia, a kā'she a, *not* a kā'se a.
acanthus, a kăn'thus, *not* ăk'an thus.
acarus, ăk'a rus, *not* a kā'rus.
acaulis, a kawl'is, *not* ăk'aw lis.
accelerator, ăk sel le rā'tor, *not* as sel'e ra tor.
acclimated, a klī'mă ted, *not* ăk'li ma ted.
accouchement, ä'kōōsh'mŏng', *not* a kōōsh'ment.
acephalus, ā sĕph'a lus, *not* a se phā'lus.

acephalic, ă sĕ phăl'ic, *not* a sĕph'a lic.
acetum, a sē'tum, *not* ăs'e tum.
acetas, a sē'tas, *not* ăs'e tas.
acetic, a sĕt'ic, *not* a sē'tic.
acetone, ăs'e tōn, *not* ă sē'tone.
acetyl, ăs'e tĭl, *not* ă sē'tĭl.
achaenium, a kē'ni um, *not* ă tchē'ni um.
achillea, ak ĭl lē'ă, *not* a kĭl'le ä.
acia, ă'shē ä, *not* ă'sē ä.
acidum, ăs'i dum, *not* a sī'dum.
acies, ă'shī ēs, *not* ă'ses.
acinus, ăs'i nus, *not* a sī'nus.
aconitum, ăk o nī'tum, *not* a kŏn'i tum.
acotyledon, a kŏt y lē'don, *not* ăk o tyl'e don.
acromion, a krō'mi on, *not* a krŏm'i on.
acyesis, a sī ē'sis, *not* a sy'e sis.
adenia, a dē'ni a, *not* ă dĕn'i a.
adeniform, a dĕn'i form, *not* a dē'ni form.
adeps, ă'dĕps, *not* ăd'eps.
adipose, ăd'i pōs, *not* ad'i pōz.
adonis, a dō'nis, *not* ă dŏn'is.
adult, ă dult', *not* ăd'ult.
adynamia, ăd ĭ nă'mi a, *not* ă dĭ năm'i a.
adynamic, ăd ĭ năm'ic, *not* ă dĭ nă'mic.
aegophony, ē gŏf'o ny, *not* ē jŏf'o ny.
aerobic, ă ē rōb'ic, *not* ē rō'bic.
aestus, ĕs'tus, *not* ēz'tus.
aetiology, ĕt i ol'ogy, *not* ē ti ol'o gy.
afferens, ăf'fe rens, *not* af fē'rens.
agamous, ăg'a mŭs, *not* a gā'mus.
agave, a gā'vē, *not* ăg'āve.
ala, ă'lä, *not* ăl'ä.
albinism, ăl'bĭ nizm, *not* ăl bī'nism.
aletris, ăl'e tris, *not* ă lē'tris.
algae, ăl'jē, *not* ăl'gē.
algoid, ăl'goid, *not* ăl'joid.

alienist, ăl′ye nist, *not* ā li c′nist.
allantoic, ăl lan tō′ic, *not* al lăn′to ic.
allantois, al lăn′to is, *not* al lăn′toy.
allopathic, ăl lo păth′ic, *not* al lŏp′a thic.
allopathy, al lŏp′a thy, *not* ăl′lo path y.
allotropic, ăl lo trŏp′ic, *not* al lŏt′ro pic.
allotropy, ăl lŏt′ro py, *not* ăl′lo trop y.
alloy, ălloy′, *not* ăl′loy.
aloe, ăl′o e, *not* ăl′ō, (Latin).
aloes, ăl′ōz, *not* ăl′ō ēz, (English).
alveolus, ăl vē′o lus, *not* ăl ve ō′lus.
amara, ā mā′ra, *not* ăm′ara.
amarin, ăm′a rin, *not* a mā′rin.
amine, ăm′ĭn or ăm′ēn, *not* ā′mĭn.
ammonia, ăm mō′ni a, *not* ā mō′ni a.
amnion, ăm′ni on, *not* ăm nī′on.
amphora, ăm′fo ra, *not* am pō′ra.
anaemic, a nĕm′ic, *not* ā nē′mic.
anaemia, a nē′mi a, *not* ā nĕm′i a.
analgesia, an al jē′si a, *not* an alge′si a.
anconeus, ăn co nē′us, *not* an cō′ne us.
anemone, a nĕm′ō nē, *not* ăn′e mōn.
anethum, a nē′thum, *not* ăn′e thum.
angina, ăn jī′nä, *not* an′gī nä.
anilin, ăn′i lĭn, *not* ăn′i lĭn.
anisum, a nī′sum, *not* ăn′i sum.
anticus, an tī′cus, *not* ăn′ti cus.
antithenar, ăn tīth′e nar, *not* an ti thē′nar.
antitragus, ăn tīt′ra gus, *not* an′ti tra gus.
anus, ā′nus, *not* ăn′us.
aphrodisiac, ā frō dīzh′i ac, *not* ăf ro dis′si ac.
aphthae, ăf′thē, *not* ăp′the.
apocynum, a pŏs′ī num, *not* ā po sy′num.
aqua, ā′kwä, *not* ăk′wä.
arabic, ăr′a bic, *not* ā rā′bic.
archebiosis, ar ke bī′ō sis, *not* ar ke bī ō′sis.

areola, á rē'o la, *not* ar e ō'la.
argemone, är jĕm'o ne, *not* är'ge mon y.
arthritis, är thrī'tis, *not* är thrē'tis.
arytenoid, a rīt'e noid, *not* ary tē'noid.
ascaris, ăs'ka ris, *not* as kä'ris.
asthenia, ăs the nī'a, *not* ăs thē'ni a.
atropa, ăt'ro pa, *not* a trō'pa.
attollens, ăt tol'lens, *not* ăt'tol lens.
atrahens, ăt'ra hens, *not* a trä'hens.
atrophic, a trŏf'ic, *not* á trō'fic.
azote, ăz'ōte, *not* ā zōt'.
azygos, ăz'ĭ gŏs, *not* a zī'gos.

B.

balanus, băl'ā nus, *not* ba lä'nus.
balsamum, băl'sa mum, *not* băwl sä'mum.
barbadoes, bär bä'dōz, *not* bär'ba dōz.
baryta, ba rī'ta, *not* băr'ĭ ta.
basilic, ba sĭl'ic, *not* băs'i lic.
bdellium, dĕl'li um, *not* be dĕl'li um.
benzoin, ben zō'in, *not* ben'zo in.
benzoinum, ben zō'i num, or ben zo i'num.
beriberi, bä rē bä'rē, *not* ber'ry berry.
bifurcate, bi fūr'cāte, *not* bi'fur cate.
bimanous, bĭm'a nus, *not* bi mä'nus.
binary, bī'na ry, *not* bĭn'a ry.
bismuth, biz'muth, *not* bĭss'muth.
biternate, bi tĕr'nate, *not* bĭt'er nate.
bitumen, bi tū'men, *not* bit'u men.
blastema, blăs tē'ma, *not* blăs'te ma.
boletus, bo lē'tus *not* bŏl'e tus.
bougie, bōō'zhē', *not* bōō jee'.
brachial, brā'ke al or brăk'e al.
brassica, brăs'si ca, *not* brăs sī'ca.
bromidum, brŏm'i dum, *not* bro mī'dum.
bronchitis, brŏng kī'tis, *not* brŏn kē'tis.

bruit, brwē, *not* brōō'y.
buchu, bōō'kōō, *not* bŭ'tchew.
butyric, bū tĭr'ic, *not* bū tī ric.
butyrin, bū'tĭ rĭn, *not* butter ēn'.

C.

cacao, cā cā'o, *not* cā'ka o.
cachexia, kā kĕx'i a, *not* kā tchĕx'i a.
cadaver, ca dā'ver, *not* cā dăv'er.
caducus, ca dū'cus, *not* căd'u cus.
caffeina, căf fe ī'nä, *not* căf fē'nä.
calabar, cal a bär', *not* căl'a ber.
calcaneum, căl cā'ne um, *not* cal ca nē'um.
caligo, cā lī'gō, *not* căl'i go.
calomelas, ca lŏm'e lās, *not* cal o mĕl'as.
caulophyllum, cawl ō phĭl'lum, *not* cau lŏph'il lum.
calor, cā'lor, *not* căl'or.
camphora, kăm'fo rä, *not* kăm fō'rä.
cancelli, kăn sĕl'lī, *not* kan'sel li.
canine, kā nīn', *not* kā'nīn nor kā nēn'.
cannabinum, kăn năb'i num, *not* kăn nā bī'num.
capillary, kăp'il la ry, preferable to ka pil'la ry.
carminative, kär mĭn'a tīve, *not* kär'mi na tive.
carotid, kā rŏt'id, *not* ka rō'tid.
caryophyllum, kär ĭ o fĭl'lum, *not* ka rĭ ōf'il lum.
cassava, căs sā'vä, *not* căs'sa vä.
cayenne, kā ĕn', *not* kī en'.
cephalic, se făl'ic, *not* sĕf'al ic.
ceratum, sē rā'tum, *not* sĕr'a tum.
cerebral, sĕr'e bral, *not* se rē'bral.
cerebrum, sĕr'e brum, *not* se rē'brum.
cerebro-spinal, sĕr'e bro-spī'nal, *not* se rē'bro-spī'nal.
cervicis, sĕr vī'cis, *not* ser'vi cis.
cervical, ser'vi cal, *not* ser vī'cal.— *Webster gives latter.*
chalazion, ka lăz'ion, *not* sha lăz'ion.
chartula, kär'tu la, *not* tchär'tu la.
6

chemosis, kē mō'sĭs, *not* tchē mō'sis.
chenopodium, kĕn o pō'dĭ um, *not* tchē no pŏd'ĭ um.
chirata, tchē rä'tä or kī rä'tä.
chiropodist, ki rŏp'o dist, *not* tchī rop'o dist.
chloridum, klor'ĭ dum, *not* klō rī'dum.
chorion, kō'ri on, *not* ko rī'on.
chorea, ko rē'a, *not* kŏr'e a.
chyle, kīl, *not* tchĭl.
chyme, kīm, *not* tchĭm.
chymification, kīm i fĭ kä'shŭn, *not* kī mi fĭ kä'shun.
cicatrix, si kä'trix, *not* si kät'rix nor sĭk'a trix.
cimicifuga, sĭm i sĭf'u gä, *not* sim i si fū'gä.
citras, sī'tras, *not* sĭt'ras.
citrate, sĭt'rate, *not* sī'trate.
clematis, klĕm'a tis, *not* kle mät'is.
cloaca, klō ä'cä, *not* klō'a cä.
cocaine, kō'ca ĭn or cō'ca ēn, *not* co cä'ĭn.
cocci, kŏk'sī, *not* kŏk'kī.
coccyx, kŏk'sĭx, *not* kŏs'sĭx.
coccygis, kŏk sī'jĭs, *not* kŏk'sī jis.
cochineal, kŏtch'ĭ nēl. *not* kō'kī nēl.
cochlea, kŏk'le a, *not* kō'kle a.
codein, kō'dē ĭn, *not* ko dē'ĭn.
codeina, kō de ĭ'nä, *not* co dī'na.
coitus, kō'i tus, *not* kō ī'tus.
comedo, kŏm'e dō, *not* ko mē'dō.
condom, kŏn'dŏm, *not* kŭn'dŭm.
conduit, kŏn'dĭt, *not* kŏn'du it.
condyle, kŏn'dĭl, *not* kŏn'dĭl.
conein, kō nē'ĭn, *not* kō'ne in.
conium, kō nī'um, *not* cō'ni um.
conjunctiva, kŏn jŭnk tī'vä, *not* kŏn junc'ti vä.
conoid, kō'noid, *not* kŏn'oid.
conserve, cŏn'serve, *not* conserve'.
contour, kōn tōōr', *not* kon'toor.
copaiba, kō pä'bä, *not* copī'bä nor co pē'bä.

coracoid, kŏr′a koid, *not* kō′ra koid.
corium, kō′ri um, *not* kō ri′um.
corolla, kō rŏl′lah, *not* kō răl′lah.
corona, ko rō′nah, *not* kŏr′o nah.
coronoid, kŏr′o noid, *not* ko rō′noid.
corpora, kŏr′pō rä, *not* kor pō′rä.
cotyledon, kot ĭ lĕ′don, *not* ko tĭl′e don,
cranium, krā′nĭ um, *not* krăn′i um.
crematory, krĕm′a tō ry, *not* krē′ma tō ry.
cricoid, krī′koid, *not* krē′koid.
crotalus, krŏt′a lus, *not* krō′ta lus.
crureus, kru rē′us, *not* krōō′re us.
cubeba, kū bē′bah, *not* ku′be bah.
culinary, kū′li nä ry, *not* kŭl′i nä ry.
cuneiform, kū′nē i form, *not* kū nē′i form.
curare, kū rä′rē or kōō rah′rä, *not* kū rä′re.
curator, kū rä′tor, *not* kūr′a tor.
cyanidum, sī ăn′i dum, *not* sī a nī′dum.
cyanosis, sī ä nō′sis, *not* sī ăn′o sis.
cyclopean, sy klō pē′an, *not* sy klŏp′e an.
cynanche, sī năng′kē, *not* sī′nä kē.
cytoblast, sīt′o blast, *not* sī′to blast.

D.

decubitus, de cū′bi tus, *not* dĕc ŭ bī′tus.
demodex, dĕm′o dex, *not* dĕ mō′dex.
dengue, däng′gä, *not* dĕng′gū.
depilatory, de pĭl′a to ry, *not* dĕp il a to ry.
deprimens, dĕp′ri mens, *not* de prī′mens.
depurant, dĕp′ū ränt, *not* dē pū′ränt.
detritus, de trī′tus, *not* dĕt′ri tus.
detrital, dĕ′tri tal, *not* de trī′tal.
diabetes, dī ä bē′tēz, *not* dē ä bĕt′es.
diabetic, dī a bĕt′ĭc, *not* di ä bē′tic.
diachylon, dī a kī′lŏn, preferable to di äk′ĭ lon.
diaphanous, dī äf′a nŭs, *not* di a fä′nŭs.

diaphragmatic, dī a frăg măt'ic, *not* di a frăm măt'ic.
diastole, dī ăs'tō le, *not* dī'ăs tōl.
diastase, dī'ăs tāz, *not* di ăs'tase.
digitalis, dǐj i tā'lis, *not* dij i tăl'is.
diphtheria, dif thē'ria, preferable to dǐp thē'ria.
diploe, dǐp'lō e, *not* dī plō'e.
discutient, dis kŭ'shent, *not* dis kū'ti ent.
distoma, dǐs'to ma, *not* di stō'ma.
dulcamara, dŭl ka mā'rah, *not* dul kăm'a rah.
duodenal, dū ŏd'e nal, *not* du o dē'nal.
duodenum, dŭ o dē'num, *not* dū ŏd'e num.
dynamite, dǐn'a mīt, *not* dī'na mīt.
dyspareunia, dǐs pa rū'ni ah, *not* dǐs pa rōō'ny.
dyspnoea, dǐsp nē'ah, *not* dǐs'ne ah.

E.

ecdysis, ĕk'dǐ sis, *not* ec dī'sis.
echinococcus, ē kī'no kok'kŭs, *not* ĕk'i no kok'kus.
ecthyma, ĕk thī'mah, *not* ĕk'thī mah.
eczema, ĕk'ze mä, *not* ĕk zē'mä.
efferens, ĕf'fe rens, *not* ĕf fē'rens.
elaterin, ē lăt'e rin, *not* ĕl a tē'rin.
elephantiasis, ĕl e phan tī'a sis, *not* el e phan ti ā'sis.
elytron, ĕl'ĭ trön, *not* e lī'tron.
embryo, ĕm'brī o, *not* em brī'o.
emesis, ĕm'e sis, *not* e mē'sis.
emmenagogne, ĕm mĕn'a gŏg, *not* ē mēn'o gawg.
emphysema, ĕm fī sē'mah or em fī zē'mah.
empyema, ĕm pī ē'mah, *not* em py ē'mi ä.
enchondroma, ĕn kŏn drō'mah, *not* en kŏn'dro mah.
endocarditis, ĕn do kär dī'tis, *not* en do kär dē'tis.
enema, ĕn'e mä, *not* e nē'mä.
enteritis, ĕn te rī'tis, *not* ĕn ter ē'tis.
entozoon, ĕn to zō'ŏn, *not* ĕn tōz'o on.
ephelis, e fē'lis, *not* ĕf'e lis.— *Thomas gives latter.*
epiphora, e pǐf'o rä, *not* ĕp i fō'rä.

epiploon, e pip'lo on, *not* ep i plō'on.
epizootic, ep i zō ŏt'ic, *not* ep i zŏŏ'tic.
epulis, e pū'lis, *not* ĕp'u lis.
ergota, er gō'tä, *not* er'go tä.
erigeron, e rĭj'e ron, *not* e righ'er on.
errhinum, ĕr rhĭ'num, *not* er rhē'num.
erythema, ĕr ĭ thē'mä, *not* erĭ thĕm'ä.
esoteric, ĕs o ter'ic, *not* e sŏt'e ric.
ethyl, ĕth'ĭl, *not* ē'thĭl.
eunuchus, ū nū'kus, *not* ū'nŏŏ kus.
eustachian, ū stä'ki an, *not* ū stätch'i an.
exanthema, ĕx an thē'mä, *not* ĕx än'the mä.
excretory. ĕx'cre to ry, preferable to ex crē'to ry.

F.

facet, făs'ĕt, *not* fä sĕt'.
facial, fā'shal, *not* făsh'al.
faradic, fa răd'ic, *not* fä rā'dic.
farcimen, fär sĭ'men, *not* fär'si men.
farina, *Lat.* fa rĭ'nah, *not* fä rē'nah.
fascia, făsh'i ah, *not* fäs'si ah.
febrile, fē'brĭl or fĕb'rĭl, *not* fē'brīl.
fetid, fĕt'id, *not* fē'tid.
fetor, fē'tor, *not* fĕt'or.
filix, fĭ'lix, *not* fē'lix.
flaccid, flăk'sid, *not* fläs'sid.
flatus, flā'tus, *not* flăt'us.
fomites, fŏm'i tēz, *not* fo mĭ'tez.
foramen, for ā'men, *not* fo răm'en.
formica, fŏr mĭ'cä, *not* for'mi cä.
fornicis, for'ni cis, *not* for nĭ'cis.
fourchette, fŏŏr'shĕt', *not* fŏŏr kĕt'.
fraxinus, frax'i nus, *not* frax ĭ'nus.
fremitus, frĕm'i tus, *not* fre mĭ'tus.
fungi, fŭn'jĭ, *not* fŭng'ghĭ.

G.

galbanum, găl'ba num, *not* gal bā'num.
gamboge, găm bōj', *not* găm'boj.
gangrene, găng'grēn, *not* găn grēn'.
gaseous, găz'e ŭs, *not* găs'se us.
gastritis, găs trī'tis, *not* găs trē'tis.
gelsemium, jel sē'mi um, *not* ghel sĕm'i um.
gelsemine, jĕl'se mĭn, *not* ghel sĕm'ēn.
gemellus, je mĕl'lus, *not* ghe mel'lus.
geranium, je rā'ni um, *not* je rĕn'i um.
gingiva, jĭn jī'vä, *not* jin'ji vä.
ginglymus, jĭng'glĭ mus, *not* ghin'gly mus.
gladiolus, gla dī'o lus, *not* glad i ō lus.
glaucoma, glaw cō'mä, *not* glow'co mä.
glenoid, glē'noid, *not* glĕn oid.
gluteus, glu tē'us, *not* glōō'te us.
gomphosis, gŏm fō'sis, *not* gŏm'fo sis.
granatum, gra nā'tum, *not* grăn'a tum.
guaiacum, gwī'a cum or gwä'ä cum, *not* gwăck'um.
gutta-percha, gŭt'tä-per tchah, *not* gutta-per'kah.

H.

hæmatemesis, hēm a tĕm'e sis, *not* hem a te mē'sis.
hæmoptysis, he mŏp'tĭ sis, *not* hē mop tī'sis.
haloid, hā loid, *not* hăl'oid.
helleborus, hĕl lĕb'o rus, *not* hel le bō'rus.
heracleum, hĕr a clē'um, *not* he răk'le um.
hiatus, hi ā'tus, *not* hī'a tus.
hippocampus, hĭp po căm pus, *not* hī po căm'pus.
hippocrates, hĭp pŏc ra tēz, *not* hī pŏc ra tez.
hippuris, hĭp pū'ric, *not* hip'pu ric.
hirsute, hir sūt, *not* her sōōt'.
hirudo, hi rū dō, *not* hir'u do.
homœopathic, hō mē o păth'ic, *not* hō mē ŏp'a thic.

homœopathy, hō mē ŏp'a thy, *not* hō'me o pathy.
hordeolum, hor dē'o lum, *not* hor de ō'lum.
humulus, hū'mū lŭs, *not* hŭm'ū lŭs.
hydatid, hī'da tid or hĭd'a tid, *not* hy dăt'id.
hydatis, hĭd'a tis, *not* hy dăt'is.
hydromel, hī'dro mel, *not* hy drŏm'el.
hydropathy, hy drŏp'a thy, *not* hī'dro path y.
hygiene, hī'gī ēn, *not* hī gēn'.
hyoides, hī oi'dēz, *not* hī'oi dēz.
hyoscyamine, hī ŏs sī'ă mĭn, *not* hy os cī ăm'ēn.
hyoscyamus, hī ŏs sī'a mus, *not* hy os sy ăm'us.
hyperinosis, hī per i nō'sis, *not* hī per īn'o sis.
hyphomyces, hī fŏm'ī sēz, *not* hī fo mī'sēz.
hypochondriasis, hi po kŏn drī'a sis, *not* hy po kŏn dri ă'sis.
hypospadias, hī po spā'di as, *not* hī po spăd'i as.

I.

iatria, i a trī'ä, *not* i ăt'ria.
ichor, ī'kŏr, *not* ĭk'ŏr.
ichthyosis, ĭk thī ō'sis, *not* ĭk thī'o sis.
icteric, ĭk tĕr'ic, *not* ĭk'ter ic.
icterus, ĭk'te rus, *not* ĭk tē'rus.
ileus, ĭl'e us, *not* i lē'us.
impetigo, ĭm pe tī'gō, *not* ĭm pĕt'i go.
impotence, ĭm'pō tence, *not* ĭm pō'tence.
infusum, in fū'sum, *not* in fū'zum.
ingluvin, ĭn'glū vĭn, *not* ĭn glū vin.
integral, ĭn'te grăl, *not* in te'gral.
intertrigo, ĭn ter trī'go, *not* in ter tri go.
intestinal, in tĕs'ti nal, *not* in tes tī'nal.
intestine, ĭn tĕs'tĭn, *not* in tĕs'tĭn.
intestinum, ĭn tes tī'num, *not* in tĕs ti num.
inula, ĭn'ū lah, *not* in ū'la.
iodidum, i ŏd'i dum, *not* i o dī'dum.
iodoform, i ŏd'o form, *not* i ō'do form.
iodum, i ō'dum, *not* ī'o dum.

ipecac, ĭp'e căc, *not* ĕp'ĭ căc.
isinglass, ī'zing glăs, *not* ī'sin glăs.
isomeric, ĭs o mer'ic, *not* ī sŏm'e ric.
isomerism, ī sŏm'ĕr izm, *not* ĭs o mē'rizm.

J.

jaborandi, zhä bō răn'dĕ, *not* jăb'o răn'dī.
jalapa, ja lä'pä, *not* jăl'a pä.
jasminum, jăs'mĭ num, *not* jas mī'num.
jaundice, jän'dĭs, *not* jawn'dis.
jejunum, jĕ jū'num, *not* jĕj'ōō num.
juglans, jū'glănz, *not* jŭg'lanz.
jugular, jū'gū lar, *not* jŭg'ular.
juniperus, jū nĭp'e rŭs, *not* ju ni pē'rus.

K.

kamala, ka mä'lä or kä mä lä, *not* kä mäl'ä.
keloid, kē'loid, *not* kĕl'oid.
keratitis, kĕr a tī'tis, *not* kĕr a tē'tis.
kino, kī'no, *not* kē'no.
kyestein, kī ĕs'te in, *not* kī'es tēn.

L.

lacteal, lăc'te al, *not* lac tē'al.
lagopus, la gō'pus, lăg'o pus.
lamella, la mĕl'lä, *not* lăm'el la.
lanthanum, lăn'tha num, *not* lăn thăn'um.
laryngectomy, lăr ĭn jĕc'tō my, *not* lar yng ghĕc'to my.
laudanum, law'dä num or lŏd'a num, *not* lawd'num.
lecethin, lĕs'e thin, *not* le sē'thin.
legumine, le gū'mĭn, *not* lĕg'ū min.
leuchæmia, lū kē'mi a, *not* lū sē'mia, unless spelled leucaemia.

lentigo, lĕn tī′gō, *not* lĕn′ti go.
levator, lĕ vä′tör, *not* le văt′or.
lientery, lī′ĕn te ry, *not* lī ĕn′te ry.
limonis, (*gen.*) li mō′nis, *not* lĭm′o nis.
Linæan, li nē′än, *not* lĭn′e an.
linea, lĭn′e ah, *not* li nē′ah.
liquor, lī′kwör, *not* lĭk′ör.
lithotripsy, lĭth′o trip sī, *not* li thŏt′riɔ sy.
lithotrity, li thŏt′ri ty, *not* lĭth′o tri ty.
lobelin, lŏb′e lĭn, *not* lo bē′lĭn.
lobulus, lŏb′ū lŭs, *not* lō′bū lus.
lordosis, lör dō′sis, *not* lör′do sis.
lumbricus, lŭm brī′cŭs, *not* lŭm′bri cus.
luteum, lū′te um, *not* lu tē′um.
lupinus, lū pī′nus, *not* lōōp′i nus.
lycopodium, lī kō pō′di um, *not* lĭk o pŏd′i um.
lycopus, lī kō′pus, *not* lĭk′o pus.
lyra, lī′rah, *not* lĭr′ah.
lysis, lī′sis, *not* lĭs′is.

M.

machina, mäk′i nah, *not* mä shē′nah.
macula, măk′ū lah, *not* ma kū′lah.
magistery, măj′is te ry, *not* ma jis′te ry.
magistral, măj′is tral, *not* ma jis′tral.
malar, mä′lär, *not* măl′är.
malleolus, măl lē′o lus, *not* mal le ō′lus.
malpighian, măl pīgh′i an, *not* măl pīj′i an.
mammillary, măm′mil la ry, *not* ma mil la ry.
manganum, măn′gä num, *not* măn gä′num.
marjoram, mär′jō răm, *not* mär jō′ram.
masseter, măs sē′ter, *not* măs′se ter.
mastiche, măs′ti kē, *not* măs′ti tchē.
mastitis, măs tī′tis, *not* mas tē′tis.
matico, mä tī′kō or mä tē′kō, *not* măt′i co.

matrix, mā'trix, *not* măt'rix.
maxillary, măk'sil la ry, *not* mak zil'la ry.
meatus, mē ā'tus, *not* me ăt'us.
meconin, mĕk'o nĭn, *not* mē kō'nĕn.
mediastinum, me di ăs tī'num, *not* me di ăs'ti num.
medullary, mĕd'ul lā ry, *not* me dŭl'la ry.
megrim, mē'grĭm, *not* mē grĭm'.
melæna, me lē'nah, *not* mĕl'e nah.
mellitus, mĕl lī'tus, *not* mĕl'li tus.
membrana, mĕm brā'nah, *not* mĕm'brā nah.
membranous, mĕm'bra nous, *not* mem brā'nous.
menstruum, men'strū ŭm, *not* mĕn'strŭm.
mephitic, mē phĭt'ic, *not* me phī'tic.
mesmerism, mĕz'mer izm, *not* mes'mer ism.
metabolic, mĕt a bŏl ic, *not* mē tăb'o lic.
meatbolism, me tăb'o lizm, *not* met a bŏl'izm.
metamorphosis, mĕt a mŏr'fō sis, (English), or metamor-
    fō'sis, (Latin).
methyl, mĕth'ĭl, *not* mē'thĭl.
metritis, mē trī'tis, *not* mĕt rē'tis.
metric, mĕt'ric, *not* mē'tric.
mezereum, mĕz e rē'um, *not* me zĕr'e um.
microscope, mī'krō skōp, *not* mĭk'rō scōp.
microscopy, mī krŏs'ko py, *not* mī'krō skō py.
microsporon, mi krŏs'po ron or mī krō spō'ron.
mimosa, mī mō'sah, *not* mĭm'o sa.
mistura, mĭs tū'rah, *not* mĭst'ū ra.
modiolus, mo dī'o lus, *not* mŏd i ō'lus.
molecule, mŏl'e kūl, *not* mō'le kŭl.
molimen, mō lī'men, *not* mŏl'i men.
molybdenum, mo lĭb dē'num, *not* mo lĭb'de num.
monad, mŏn'ad, *not* mō'nad.
monomania, mŏn ō mā'ni a, *not* mō nō mā'ni a.
morphine, mor'phĭn or mor'fēn, *not* mor fēn'.
morphœa, mor fē'ah, *not* mor'fe ah.
mucilago, mū si lā'go, *not* mu sĭl'a go.

muscari, mŭs kä'rĭ, *not* mŭs'ka ri.
muscarine, mŭs'kä rĭn, *not* mŭs kä'rēn.
musci, mŭs'sĭ, *not* mŭs'kĭ.
myselium, mĭ sē'li um, *not* mĭ sēl'ĭ um.
myoides, mĭ oi'dēz, *not* mĭ'oi dēz.
myoma, my ō'mah, *not* mĭ'o mah.
myrrha, mĭr'rhah, *not* mer'rhä.
myxœdema, mĭx ē dē'mah, *not* mĭx ĕd'e mah.

N.

nana, nä'nah, *not* nän'ah.
narceina, när sē ĭ'nah, *not* när sĭ'nah.
nascent, näs'sent, *not* nä'sent.
nates, nä'tēz, *not* nät'ēz.
nematodes, nĕm a tō'dēz, *not* nĕm'ä tōds.
nephritis, nē frĭ'tis, *not* nĕ frē'tis.
neurasthenia, nūr äs the nĭ'ah, *not* nūr äs thē'ni ah.
neuroglia, nū rŏg'li ah, *not* neu rō gli'ah.—*Thomas gives latter.*
nomenclature, no men'kla tūr, *not* no'men cla ture.
nosology, nō sŏl'o gy, *not* no zŏl'o gy.
nubile, nū'bĭl, *not* nōō'bĭl.
nucha, nū'kah, *not* nōōt'cha.
nucleolus, nū klē'o lus, *not* nū klē ō'lus.
nymphæan, nĭm fē'än, *not* nĭm'fe an.
nystagmus, nĭs täg'mus, *not* nĭ stäg'mus.

O.

obesity, ō bĕs'ĭ ty, *not* ō bē'si ty.
obliquus, o blĭk'wŭs, *not* ŏb lĭ'kwus nor ob lē'kwus.
obovate, ŏb ō'väte, *not* ŏb'o väte.
obturator, ŏb tū rä'tor, *not* ŏb'tū rät'or.
obverse, ŏb'verse, *not* ŏb vers'.
ocimum, ō sĭ'mum, *not* ŏs'ĭ mum.

œdema, ē dē'mah, *not* ē dĕm'ah.
œdematous, ē dĕm'a tŭs, *not* ē dē'ma tŭs.
œstrum, ēs'trum, *not* ē'strum.
officina, ŏf fi sī'nah, *not* ŏf fĭs'i nah.
officinal, ŏf fĭs'i nal, *not* ŏf fi sī'nal.
oleomargarine, ō lē ō mär'gâ rĭn, *not* ō lē ō mär'jä rēn.
oleoresina, ō lē ō re zī'nah, *not* o le o rĕz'i nah.
oliva, ō lī'vah, *not* ŏl'i vah.
omasum, ō mā'sum, *not* ŏm'a sum.
oophorectomy, ō ŏ fō rĕk tō mī, *not* ŏp or ĕk'to my.
ophiasis, ō fī'ä sis, *not* ŏf i ä sis.
ophthalmic, ŏf thäl'mic, *not* ŏp thäl'mic.
opponens, ŏp pō'nens, *not* ŏp'pō nens.
orchitis, or kī'tis, *not* or kē'tis.
origanum, ō rĭg'a num, *not* or ij ä'num.
orthopedic, ŏr thō pĕd'ic, *not* or thŏ pē'dic.
oryza, ō rī'zah, *not* or'ĭ zah.
osmazome, ŏs'mä zōme, *not* ŏs mä'zome.
osmosis, ŏs mō'sis, *not* ŏs'mo sis.
osteoid, ŏs'tē oĭd, *not* ŏs'toid.
ovale, ō vä'le, *not* ō väl'e.
oxalic, ŏk säl'ic, *not* ŏk sal ic.
oxalis, ŏk'sa lis, *not* ŏk säl'is.
oxide, ŏk'sĭd, *not* ŏk'sīd.
oxytocic, ŏk sī tŏs'ic, *not* oxy tŏk'ic nor oxy tŏx'ic.
ozæna, ō zē'nah, *not* ō zĕn'ah.
ozone, ō'zōn, *not* ō zōn'.

P.

pacini, pä tchē'nē, *not* pa sī'nī.
pacinian, pä sĭn'i an, *not* pä tchĕn'i an.
pædiatry, pĕd i a trī, *not* pē'di a try.
pædiatrics, pĕd i ät'rĭks, *not* pē di ät'riks.
palatine, päl'a tĭn, *not* päl'ä tĭn.
palatum, pa lä'tum, *not* päl'a tum.
paliative, päl'i a tĭv, *not* päl'a tĭv.

palmaris, pål mä'ris, *not* pål'ma ris.
palpebra, pål'pē brah, *not* pål pē'brah.
paludal, pa lū'dal, *not* pål u dal.
panacea, păn a sē'ah, *not* pa nä'se a.
pancreatin, păn'krē a tĭn, *not* păn krē'a tĭn.
panis, pā'nis, *not* păn'is.
papaver, pā pā'ver, *not* påp'a ver.
papyrus, pā pī'rus, *not* påp'y rus.
paracentesis, pår a sen tē'sis, *not* par ā sĕn'te sis.
parasitic, pår a sĭt'ic, *not* par a si tic.
pareira brava, pā rī rah brā'vah, *not* pā rē rah bräv a.
parenchyma, pår ĕn'kĭ mah, *not* par ĕn kĭ'mah.
parenchymatous, pår ĕn kĭm'a tŭs, *not* par en kĭ'ma tŭs.
paresis, pår'ē sis, *not* pā rē'sis.
paretic, pā rĕt'ic, *not* pā rē tic.
parietal, pā rī'e tal, *not* pår i ē'tål.
paronychia, pår o nĭk'i a, *not* par o nitch'i a.
parotid, pa rŏt'id, *not* pā rō'tid.
partridge-berry, pär'tridj-ber ry, *not* påt'ridj-ber ry.
pathogenic, påth o jĕn'ic, *not* pā thŏj'e nic.
pathogeny, pā thŏj'e ny, *not* path o gē ny.
pectoral, pĕk'tō ral, *not* pĕk tō'ral.
pedal, (*adj.*) pē'dal, *not* pĕd'al.
peduncle, pē dŭnk'le, *not* pē'dunk le.
pellagra, pĕl'la grah, *not* pĕl läg'rah.
pemphigus, pĕm'fi gus, *not* pem fi'gus.
pepo, pē'pō, *not* pĕp'o.
pepsinum, pĕp sī'num, *not* pĕp'si num.
perinaeum, per i nē'um, *not* pe rin'e um.
peristaltic, per i stål'tic, *not* per i stawl'tic.
peritonitis, per i tō nī'tis, *not* per i tō nē'tis.
peroneus, per ō nē'ŭs, *not* per ō'ne ŭs.
petal, pĕt'al or pē'tal.
peyer, pī'er, *not* pā'er.
phagedaena, făj ē dē'nah, *not* făj e dĕn'ah.
phagedenic, făj e dĕn'ic, *not* făj e dē'nic.

pharmaceutic, fär ma sū'tic, *not* fär mā kū'tic.
pharmacopœa, fär ma kō pē'ah, *not* fär mā kō'pe ah.
phenic, fĕn'ic, *not* fē'nic.
phrenic, frĕn'ic, *not* frē'nic.
phthisis, tī'sis or thī'sis, *not* tē'sis,
phylloxera, fĭl lŏk sē'rah, *not* fĭl lŏk'se rah.
physostigma, fĭs ō stĭg'mah, *not* fī sō stĭg'mah.
phytosis, fi tō'sis, *not* fĭt'o sis.
pilocarpus, pĭl o kär'pŭs, *not* pī lo kar'pus.
pilula, pĭl'ū lah, *not* pi lōō'lah.
pineal, pĭn'e al, *not* pī'ne al.
pisiform, pĭs'si form or pĭz'i form, *not* pē'zi form.
pityriasis, pi tĭ rī'a sis, *not* pi tĭ ri ā'sis.
plantago, plăn tā'gō, *not* plăn'ta go.
platinum, plăt'i num or pla tī'num.
platysma, plā tĭs'mah, *not* plăt'ĭs mah.
podagra, pŏd'a grah, pō dăg'ra *sometimes given.*
podophylline, pŏd ō fĭl'lĭn, *not* po dŏf'ĭl lĕn.
podophyllum, pŏd ō fĭl'lum, *not* pō dŏf'ĭl lum.
polygala, pō lĭg'a lah, *not* pŏl ĭ gā'lah.
polygonum, pō lĭg ō'num, *not* pŏ ly gō'num.
porrigo, por rī'go, *not* por'rĭ gō.
posterior, pŏs tē'ri or, *not* pōs tē'ri or.
posticus, pŏs tī'cus, *not* pōs'ti cus.
posthumous, pŏst'hū mŭs, *not* pōst hū'mŭs.
prepuce, prē'pŭs, *not* prĕp'ōōs.
preventive, prē vĕn'tĭv, *not* pre vĕn'ta tĭv.
process, prŏ'sĕs, *not* prō'sĕs.
protean, prō'te an, *not* prō tē'an.
prurigo, prū rī'go, *not* prōōr'i go.
pruritus, prū rī'tus, *not* prōōr'ri tus.
psammodes, săm mō'dēz, *not* săm'ō dĕz.
pterygium, te rĭj'i um, tē rĭgh'ĭ um.
pterygoid, ter'ĭ goid, *not* ter'ĭ joid.
ptomaine, tō'mā ĭn, *not* tō'mĭn nor to mān'.
puerile, pū'er ĭl, *not* pū'er īl.

purpura, pŭr'pū rah, *not* pŭr pū'rah.
purulent, pū'rū lent, *not* pŭr ōō lent.
pygmean, pĭg mē'an, *not* pĭg'me an.
pyriform, pĭr'i form, *not* pĭ ri form.
pyrethrum, pĭr'e thrum, *not* pĭ rē'thrum.
pyrites, pĭ rī'tēz, *not* pī'ri tēz.
pyrosis, pĭ rō'sis, *not* pīr'o sis.
pyrus, pī'rus, *not* pĭr'us.

Q.

quadrumana, kwäd rōō'ma nä, *not* kwäd ru mä'nä.
quassia, kwäsh'i a or kwŏsh'i a, *not* kwäs si a.
quaternary, kwä'ter na ry, *not* kwä ter'na ry.
quebracho, kä brä tchō, *not* kwē bräk'o.
quinate, kwī'nāt, *not* kwĭn'āt.
quinina, kwĭ nī'nah, *not* kwĭ nē'nah.
quinine, kwī'nīn, kwī'nĭn or kwĭ nīn', *not* kwĭ nēn'.

R.

rabies, rā'bĭ ēz, *not* răb'i ēz.
rhachitis, rä kī'tis, rä kē'tis.
radix, rā'dix, *not* răd'ix.
rale, räl, *not* răl.
raphe, rā'fē, *not* rä fā'.
raspberry, răz'ber ry, *not* răs'berry nor raws'berry.
reflex, (*noun.*) rē'flĕx, *not* rē flex'.
renal, rē'nal, *not* rĕn al.
reniform, rĕn'i form, *not* rē'ni form.
resina, re zī'nah, *not* rĕz'i nah.
resorcin, rē zōr'sĭn, *not* rĕz'or sin.
retrahens, rĕt'ra hens, *not* rē trä'hens.
rhinoplasty, rĭn'o plăs ty, *not* rī'no plăs ty.
rhizoma, ri zō'mah, *not* rīz'o mah.
rhoncus, rŏng'kŭs, *not* rŏn'kŭs.
ricinus, rĭs'i nus, *not* ri sī'nus.

rigor, rī'gor, *not* rĭg'or.
roseola, ro zē'o lah, *not* rō zē ō lah.
rostellate, rŏs'tĕl lāt, *not* rō stĕl'lāt.
rubedo, ru bē'do, *not* rū'be do.
rubeola, ru bē'ō lah, *not* ru bē ō'lah.
rubigo, ru bī'go, *not* rū'bĭ go.
rugae, ru'jē, *not* rōō'ghē.
rupia, ru'pi ah, *not* ru pī'ah.

S.

sabbatia, săb bā'shē a, *not* sā băt'ti a.
saccharum, săk'kā rum, *not* săk kā'rum.
sacrum, sā'krum, *not* săk'rum.
sagittal, săj'ĭt tal, *not* sā jĭt'tal.
salicylic, săl ĭ sĭl'ic, *not* săl sĭl'ic.
saline, sā lĭn', *not* sā'lĭn nor sā'lēn.
salivary, săl'ĭ vā ry, *not* sā lĭ'va ry.
salix, sā'lix, *not* săl'ix.
sambucus, săm bū'cŭs, *not* săm'bŭk ŭs.
santalum, săn'tā lum, *not* san tā'lum.
sarcina, săr sī'nah, *not* săr'sī nah.
sativa, sa tī'vah, *not* sā tē'vah.
saturnine, săt'ur nĭn, *not* sā tŭr'nĕn.
satyriasis, sa tĭ rī'a sis, *not* săt ĭr i ā'sis.
saxifraga, săk sif'rā gah, *not* săk si frā'gah.
scabies, ska'bĭ ēz, *not* skāb'ĕz.
scalenus, ska lē'nŭs, *not* skăl'e nus.
scalpel, skăl'pĕl, *not* skăl pĕl'.
scarlatina, scär la tī'nah or scär la tē'nah, (Italian).
schindylesis, skĭn dĭ lē'sis, *not* shĭn dĭl'e sis.
schizomycetes, skĭz ō mi sē'tēz, *not* shiz o mĭ'sē tes.
scilla, sĭl'lah, *not* skĭl'lah.
scirrhus, skĭr'rŭs, *not* shĭr'rus.
scybalous, sĭb'ā lŭs, *not* skĭb'a lŭs.
secale, sē kā'lē, *not* sē kăl'e.
sempervirens, sĕm per'vĭ renz, *not* sĕm per vī'rens.

senna, sĕn'nah, *not* sē'nah.
sequelæ, sē kwē'lē, *not* sĕk'wē lē.
sialagogue, sī ăl'ă gŏg, *not* sē ăl'ō gawg.
sinapis, si nă'pis, *not* sīn'ă pis.
sinapism, sĭn'ă pizm, *not* sī'nă pizm.
solanum, sō lă'num, *not* sōl'ă num.
sorghum, sor'gum, *not* sŏr'jum.
spermaceti, sper mă sē'tī, *not* sper mă sĕt'i.
sphenoid, sfē'noid, *not* sfēn'oid.
sphygmograph, sfĭg'mō grăf, *not* smĭg'mo grăf.
splenic, splĕn'ic, *not* splē'nic.
spongoid, spŏng'goid, *not* spŭn'joid.
squamous, skwā'mŭs, *not* skwăm'ŭs nor skwă'mus.
static, stăt'ic, *not* stā'tic.
strangury, străng'gū ry, *not* străn'jū ry.
suberic, sū ber'ic, *not* sŭb'a ric.
sublimis, sŭb lī'mĭs, *not* sŭb'li mis.
subsidence, sŭb sī'dents, *not* sŭb'sī dents.
succinic, sŭk sĭn'ic, *not* sŭs'i nic.
succinum, sŭk'sī num, *not* sŭk sī'num.
sulphurous, sŭl'fū rŭs, *not* sŭl fū'rŭs.
suppurate, sŭp'pū rāt, *not* sŭp'per ăt.
sutura, sū tū'rah, *not* sōōt'u rah.
synechia, sĭn ē kī'a, *not* sĭn etch'i a.
synizesis, sĭn ĭ zē'sis, *not* sĭn ĭz'e sis.
synovitis, sĭn ō vī'tis, *not* sī nō vē'tis.
syphilides, sĭ fĭl'ĭ dēz, *not* sĭf'ĭ lĭdz.
syringe, (*noun.*) sĭr'inj, *not* sŭr inj'.
syrupus, sĭ rū'pŭs, *not* sur'ŭ pus.
systema, sĭs tē'mah, *not* sĭs'te mah.
systemic, sĭs tĕm'ic, *not* sĭs tē'mic.
systole, sĭs'tō lē, *not* sĭs'tōl.

T.

tabacum, to bă'kum, *not* tăb'a kum.
tabes, tă'bēz, *not* tăb'ēz.
7

tartaric, tär tär'ic, *not* tär tär ic.
taurin, taw'rĭn, *not* tow'rin.
telluric, tel lu'ric, *not* tĕl'lu ric.
terebinthina, ter e bĭn'thĭ nah, *not* ter e bĭn thĭ'nah.
tetanic, te tăn'ic, *not* tĕt'ā nic.
tetanoid, tĕt'a noid, *not* te tăn'oid.
tetrad, tĕt'răd, *not* tĕ'trad.
thalamus, thăl'a mus, *not* tha lă'mus.
thyme, tĭm, *not* thĭm.
thymus, thĭ'mŭs, *not* tī'mŭs.
tinctura, tĭnk tū'rah, *not* tink'tōō rah.
tinea, tĭn'e ah, *not* tĭn ē'a.
tinnitus, tĭn nī'tus, *not* tĭn'ni tus.
thracelo-mastoid, trā kĕ'lo-măs'toid, *not* trăk'ē lō-măs'toid.
trachoma, tra kŏ'mah, *not* trăk'ō mah.
tragacanth, trăg'a kanth, *not* trăj'i canth.
tremor, trĕ'mor, *not* trĕm'or.
trichiasis, tri kī'a sis, *not* trĭk i ā'sis.
trichina, trī kī'nah, *not* trī kĕ'nah.
tricolor, trĭk'ō lor, *not* trī'kō lor.
trigone, trī'gōn or trĕ'gōn, (French), *not* trī'gawn.
tripartite, trī'pär tīt, *not* trī pär tīt.
triquetra, trī kwĕ'trah, *not* trĭk'ē trah.
troche, trō'kĕ, *not* trō'tchee nor trōtch.
trochisci, trō kĭs'sī, *not* trō kis'kī.
trochlea, trŏk'lē ah, *not* trō'kle ah.
turpethum, tŭr'pē thum, *not* tŭr pē'thum.
tympanum, tĭm'pa num, *not* tĭm păn'um.
tyrosin, tĭr'ō sĭn, *not* tī'rō sĭn.
tyrotoxicon, tĭr ō tŏk'sĭ kon, *not* tī rō tŏk'si kon.

U.

umbellate, ŭm'bĕl lāt, *not* ŭm bĕl'lāt.
umbilicus, ŭm bĭ li'cus, *not* ŭm bĭl'i cus.—*Webster gives latter.*
unguentum, ŭng gwĕn'tum, *not* ŭn gwĕn'tum.

unguinal, ŭng′gwĭ nal, *not* ŭn gwē′nal.
urachus, ū′rā kŭs, *not* ū răk′ŭs.
uræmic, ŭr rĕm′ĭc, *not* ŭ rē′mĭc.
uredo, ū rē′do, *not* ū′rĕ dō.
ureter, ū rē′ter, preferable to ū′re ter.
urethra, ū rē′thra, *not* ū′re thra.
urtica, ŭr tĭ′cah, *not* ŭr′ti can.
ustilago, ŭs tĭ lă′go, *not* ŭs til′a go.
uterine, ū′ter ĭn, *not* ū′ter ĭn.

V.

vaccina, văk sĭ′nah, *not* văk′sĭ nah.
vagina, va jĭ′nah, *not* văj′i nah.
vaginal, văj′i nal, *not* vā jĭ′nal.
variola, vă rĭ′ō lah, *not* văr i ō′lah.
varioloid, văr′i ō loid, *not* văr ĭ ō loid′.
vena, vē′nah, *not* vā′nah.
venereal, ve nē′re al, *not* vĕn′e ral.
veratrum, vē rā′trum, *not* vē răt′rum.
veronica, vē rō nĭ′cah, preferable to ve rŏn′i cah.
vertebral, ver′te bral, *not* ver.tē′bral.
verruca, ver rū′kah, *not* vē rŭk′kah.
versicolor, ver sĭk′o lor, *not* ver′si cō lor.
verumontanum, vē ru mŏn tā′num, *not* vē ru mŏn′ta num.
vesica, vē sĭ′kah, *not* vĕs′i kah.
vesical, vĕs′i căl, *not* vē sĭ′cal.
vesicle, vĕs′i kl, *not* vē′si kl.
veterinary, vĕt′er i nā ry, *not* vē ter′i na ry.
vibriones, vĭb ri ō′nēz, *not* vĭ′bri ō nez.
vieussens, vē′ūs′sŏng′, *not* vĭ ūs′ĕnz.
viola, vī′ō lah, *not* vi ō′la.
vitelline, vī tĕl′lĭn, *not* vĭt′el lĕn.
vomitus, vŏm′i tŭs, *not* vo mĭ′tus.
vulgaris, vŭl gā′ris, *not* vŭl găr′is.

W. X. Y. Z.

wintera, wĭn tĕ'rah, *not* wĭn'tĕ rah.

xiphoid, zĭf'oid, *not* zī'foid.

yolk, yōlk, *not* yĕlk.

zoology, zō ŏl'ō jy, *not* zōō ŏl'ō jv.

zygoma, zy gō'mah, *not* zig'ō mah.

zygomatic, zĭg ō măt'ic.

CHAPTER IV.

THERE are eight parts of speech in Latin, four of which, *nouns, adjectives, pronouns* and *verbs*, are inflected, while the other four, *adverbs, prepositions, conjunctions* and *interjections*, remain unchanged.

By *inflection* we mean the change of form which words undergo to denote their relation to other words. These changes are much more numerous and complicated in Latin and Greek than in English, and great care must be taken to learn them accurately. In English the meaning of a sentence depends largely upon the arrangement of the words. This, however, is not the case with inflectional languages, for in these nearly all relations are expressed by inflections or terminations; thus, *Josephus os cani dat*, may be translated, "Joseph a bone to the dog gives;" *Josepho os cani datur*, "By Joseph a bone to the dog is given."

This latter sentence might also have the words arranged in any other order, but the usual method is to place the subject first, the object second, and the predicate last.

1. That variety of inflection which nouns, adjectives and participles undergo is called *declension*. By declension we express the gender, number and case of words.

2. There are three genders in Latin as in English, the masculine, feminine and neuter, but these have little to do with sex, as we understand it. The ancients believed sex to be an inherent quality in all objects, as at a later period we found the alchemists believing that metals were of various sexes.

3. *Number.* There are two numbers in Latin as in English.

4. *Cases.* There are six cases in Latin, viz.:—

(*a*) The *nominative*, used as in English.

(*b*) The *genitive*, denoting origin, possession or partition.

(*c*) The *dative*, denoting that to or for which a thing is done.

(*d*) The *accusative*, almost equivalent to the English objective.

(*e*) The *vocative*, used in addressing persons or things.

(*f*) The *ablative*, denoting the relation expressed in English by *from, with, by*, or *in*.

In the following sentence all the cases will be found: *Josephe (voc.), det Henricus (nom.) os (accusative) ovis (gen.) cani (dat.) sylva (abl.)*, Joseph (*voc.*) let Henry (*nom.*) give a bone (*acc.*) of a sheep (*gen.*) to the dog (*dat.*) from the woods (*abl.*)

There are five declensions in Latin, distinguished by the endings of the genitive singular. The following table contains nearly all the case endings arranged according to declensions.

SINGULAR.

DECLENSIONS.	I.	II.	III.	IV.	V.
CASE.					
Nominative.	a (e)	us, es, um	es, is, or, etc.	us, u	es
Genitive	æ	i	is	us	ei
Dative	æ	ō	i	ûi, u	ei
Accusative..	am	um	em, im, etc.	um, u	em
Vocative ...	a	e, um	like Nom.	us, u	es
Ablative	â	ō	e or i	u	e

PLURAL.

DECLENSIONS.	I.	II.	III.	IV.	V.
CASE.					
Nominative.	æ	i, a	es, a	us, ûa	es
Genitive	a'rum	ö'rum	um, lum	ûum	e'rum
Dative......	is	is	ibus	ibus, ûbus	e'bus
Accusative..	as	os, a	es, a	us, ûa	es
Vocative....	æ	i, a	es, a	us, ûa	es
Ablative	is	is	ibus	ibus, ûbus	e'bus

CHAPTER V.

The First Declension.

NOUNS of the first declension usually end in *a*. They are all feminine except such as denote males.

Costa, a rib, is declined as follows : —

	SINGULAR.	PLURAL.
Nom.	cost a, a rib	cost ae, ribs
Gen.	cost ae, of a rib	cost a'rum, of ribs
Dat.	cost ae, to or for a rib	cost is, to or for ribs
Acc.	cost am, a rib	cost as, ribs
Voc.	cost a, O rib	cost ae, O ribs
Abl.	cost a, by, with, or from a rib	cost is, by, with, or from ribs

VOCABULARY I.

aca'cia, æ (fr. Greek ἀκή, a prickle) acacia.

ala, æ (contraction of *axilla*) a wing, side.

an'ima, æ (fr. ἄνεμος, the wind) air, vital principle.

angi'na, æ (fr. *ango*, Greek ἄγχω, to strangle) sore throat, quinsy.

aura, æ (cf. Greek αὔω, to blow) a break of air, premonition.

auric'ula, æ (dim. of *auris*, an ear) a small ear, auricle.

bacca, æ (——————) a berry.

bulla, æ (fr. *bullio*, to boil) a bubble, a lump, ball.

bursa, æ (fr. Greek βύρσα. the hide of an ox, βοῦς) a leather pouch, a purse.

braye'ra, æ (fr. Dr. Brayer, a French botanist) kooso.

bryo'nia, æ (fr. βρύω, to grow luxuriantly) bryony.

coro'na, æ (fr. Greek κορώνη, a garland) a crown.

chimaph'ila, æ (fr. Greek χεῖμα, winter, and φιλέω, to love) pipsissewa.

cor'nea, æ (fr. *cornu*, a horn) the cornea.

fari'na æ (fr. *far*, a kind of grain) meal, flour.

fas'cia, æ (cf. *fascis*, a bundle) a bandage, a fibrous membrane.

fib'ula, æ (cf. *fibulo*, to clasp) a buckle tongue, a brace, fibula, also an instrument used by the Romans for stitching the *labia majora*, or the prepuce in the male, to prevent copulation.

fis'tula, æ (cf. *fistuca*, a rammer) a pipe, tube, fistula.

fossa, æ (fr. *fodio*, to dig) a ditch, trench, groove.

gemma, æ (cf. Greek γέμω, to swell up) a bud.

gutta, æ (perhaps allied to *gusto*, to taste) a drop.

althæ'a, æ (Greek ἄλθω, to heal) marsh mallow.

amen'tia, æ (*a* without, *mens*, mind) total loss of mind.

ampul'la, æ (*ambi*, about *olla*, a pot) a two handled jug or jar.

angustu'ra, æ (*Angostura*, a town in Venezuela) a bitter plant.

anten'na, æ (fr. *ante*, before, and *teneo*, to hold, lit. a yard-arm or end rope) the "feelers" of insects.

aqua, æ (cf. *equalis*, level) water.

ar'nica, æ (fr. Greek ἀρς, a lamb, fr. the soft leaf) arnica.

artemis'ia, æ (fr. *Artemis*, Greek Ἄρτεμις, Diana) a plant.

ave'na, æ (*a*, without, *vena*, vein) oats.

cap'sula, æ (dim. of *capsa*, a box) small box, capsule.

cera, æ (Greek κηρός, wax) bleached wax.

char'tula, æ (dim. of *charta*, a parchment) a powder paper.

cimicif'uga, æ (fr. *cimex*, a bug, and *fugo*, to put to flight) black-snake root.

chorda, æ (χορδή, a cord made of intestine) a cord.

et, and.

EXERCISE I.

A 1. Guttae aquae. 2. Fistula corneae. 3. Gemmae et baccae. 4. Aqua ammoniae. 5. Fossae costarum. 6. Corona et alae. 7. Aura epilepsiae. 8. Bullae et bursa. 9. Farina avenae. 10. Ampulla aquae.

B 1. The bandage of the brace (bone). 2. Buds of acacia. 3. Capsules of wax. 4. Althaea and powder papers. 5. Cords and sail ropes. 6. Chalk and water. 7. The crown of the cornea. 8. Angustura berries. 9. Sore throat and cholera. 10. A (leather bag) of water.

GREEK NOUNS OF THE FIRST DECLENSION.

A number of Greek words have been taken without much alteration into the Latin language and their declension varies from that of pure Latin nouns.

The majority of these Greek nouns end in *e* but there are a few in *es*. Those ending in *e* are feminine, the others are masculine.

Pleg′mone, from φλέγω to burn or inflame, an inflammation of cellular tissue, is declined as follows:—

	SINGULAR.	PLURAL.
Nom.	phleg′mone	phleg′monae
Gen.	phleg′mones	phlegmona′rum
Dat.	phleg′monae	phleg′monis
Acc.	phleg′monen	phleg′monas
Voc.	phleg′mone	phleg′monae
Abl.	phleg′mone	phleg′monis

In the same manner are declined all nouns ending in *cele* and such words as the following:—

acne, (supposed to a modification ἀκμή, *acme*, the prime of life, because it affects those in the bloom of youth) an eruptive skin disease.

aga′ve, (fr. ἀγαμαι, to wonder at) the century plant.

al'oe, (fr. ἀλοάω, to trample under foot) aloes.

anem'one, (fr. ἄνεμος, the wind) wind flower.

argem'one, (fr. ἀργεμον, an eye disease) thorn poppy.

daphne, (fr. Δάφνη, a river nymph changed into a bay tree) a kind of laurel.

mas'tiche, (Greek μαστίχη, fr. μαστάζω, to chew) a plant with sialagogue properties.

stat'ice, (fr. ἵστημι, to staunch) named from its astringent properties.

The Greek nouns of the first declension ending in *es* are, as a rule, declined only in the singular. *Pyri'tes* (fr. πῦρ, fire, and λίθος, stone), will serve as an example :—

Nom.	pyri'tes
Gen.	pyri'tae
Dat.	pyri'tae
Acc.	pyri'ten
Voc.	pyri'te or a
Abl.	pyri'ta or e

VOCABULARY II.

calen'dula, æ (καλένδαι, a calender, from the numerous leaves), marigold.

drach'ma, æ (Greek δραχμή, a coin), a drachm.

dulcama'ra, æ (*dulcis*, sweet; *amarus*, bitter), bittersweet.

essen'tia, æ (*ex*, out of; *ens*, participle of *esse*, to be) essence.

forma, æ (allied to μορφή, form), a shape, form.

form'ula, æ (dim. of *forma*), a small form; a set rule.

fran'gula, æ (fr. *frango*, to break), buckthorn.

galla, æ (*Gallia*), oak apple; gall nut.

gaulthe'ria, æ (fr. name of Dr. Gaulthier), wintergreen.

gena, æ (cf. Greek γένυς, cheek bone), the cheek.

glan'dula, æ (dim. of *glans*, a gland), a small gland.

hora, æ (Greek ὥρα, an hour), an hour.

ichthyocol'la, æ (fr. Greek ἰχθύς, a fish, and κόλλα, glue), isinglass.

iner'tia, æ (*in*, without; *ars*, art, activity), inactivity.

in'ula, æ (corruption of *Helenium*, fr. Helen of Troy), elecampane.

lach'ryma, æ (cf. δάκρυ, a tear), a tear.

lacu'na, æ (fr. *lacus*, a lake), a small cavity in osseous tissue.

lam'ina, æ (fr. same root as ἐλαύνω, to drive) a plate or layer.

lappa, æ (*lappa*, a clitbur), burdock.

libra, æ (cf. Greek λίτρα, a coin), a balance, a pound.

leptan'dra, æ (fr. λεπτός, slender, and ἀνήρ, stamen), Culver's root.

lin'ea, æ (cf. *linum*, flax fibre), a line.

lingua, æ (onomatopœic, fr. licking sound), the tongue.

lobe'lia, æ (fr. Lobel, a Flemish botanist), Indian tobacco.

lupuli'na, æ (fr. *lupulus*, lit. a small wolf; a name for hops), pollen from hops.

lympha, æ (lit. pure water), lymph.

mac'ula, æ (dim. fr. same root as μάχομαι, to fight), small spot on skin.

mamma, æ (Greek μάμμα, breast), breast.

massa, æ (cf. Greek μάζα, a lump of dough), a mass.

mate'ria, æ (fr. *mater*, a producer), that which is produced; matter.

maxil'la, æ (augmented fr. *mala*, cheek bone), jaw bone.

mamil'la, æ (dim. of *mamma*, the breast), the nipple.

maran'ta, æ (named in honor of *Maranti*, a Venetian botanist), arrow-root.

medici'na, æ (fr. *medeor*, to heal), the art of healing; a medicine.

medul'la, æ (fr. *medius*, middle, centre), the marrow.

membra'na, æ (fr. *membrum*, a member), a membrane.

mentha, æ (Greek μίνθη, mint), mint.

mica, æ (fr. *mico*, to sparkle like the motes in a sunbeam),
  particle; a crumb.

mistu'ra, æ (fr. *misceo*, to mix), a mixture.

mor'rhua, æ (fr. μῶρος, stupid), codfish.

mu'cuna, æ (fr. *mucus*), cowhage.

   est, is.   **sunt,** are.

EXERCISE II.

A. 1. Lacunae et medulla. 2. Libra aloes. 3. Mistura cretae. 4. Laminae fibulae. 5. Massa cerae. 6. Mistura marantae et menthae. 7. Lappa est medicina anginae. 8. Lympha et lachrymae. 9. Mistura mastiches et myrrhae. 10. Micae et galla. 11. Medulla fibulae.

B. 1. Masses, crumbs and mixtures. 2. The spots of the tongue. 3. The line of the fibula. 4. The wing of the balance. 5. The spots on the cheek in acne. 6. The lacunae of the jaw-bone.

CHAPTER VI.

THE SECOND DECLENSION.

NOUNS of the second declension end in *us*, *um*, *ir*, *er*, *os* and *on*. Those ending in *um* and *on* are neuter, the others are masculine. The great majority of the nouns of this declension used in medical works end in *us* or *um*. Those ending in *os* and *on* are of Greek origin.

Digitus, a word kindred with δείχνυμι, to point, like *indico*, is declined as follows:—

	SINGULAR.	PLURAL.
Nom.	dig′it us, a finger	dig′it i, fingers
Gen.	dig′it i, of a finger	dig it o′rum, of fingers
Dat.	dig′it o, to or for a finger	dig′it is, to or for fingers
Acc.	dig′it um, a finger	dig′it os, fingers
Voc.	dig′it e, O finger	dig′it i, O fingers
Abl.	dig′it o, by, with, or from a finger	dig′it is, by, with or from fingers

Folium, from the same root as φύλλον, a leaf, is declined as follows:—

	SINGULAR.	PLURAL.
Nom.	fo′li um, a leaf	fo′li a, leaves
Gen.	fo′li i, of a leaf	fo li o′rum, of leaves
Dat.	fo′li o, to or for a leaf	fo′li is, to or for leaves
Acc.	fo′li um, a leaf	fo′li a, leaves
Voc.	fo′li um, O leaf	fo′li a, O leaves
Abl.	fo′li o, by, with, or from a leaf	fo′li is, by, with, or from leaves

VOCABULARY III.

ac'inus, i (Greek ἄκινος, a grape), a granule; kernel; part of a gland.

alve'olus, i (dim. of *alvus,* the belly), a little belly, cavity, socket.

an'imus, i (ἄνεμος, the wind), the mind, soul.

an'nulus, i (dim. of *annus,* a circle, a ring), a little ring.

anus, i (fr. *annus,* a ring; cf. ἀμφί, around), orifice of rectum.

bacil'lus, i (dim. of *baculum,* a staff), a little rod; rod-like bacterium.

bolus, i (Greek βῶλος, a clod), a lump, mouthful, large pill.

bulbus, i (Greek βολβός, an onion), a bulb.

cal'amus, i (Arabic *kalam,* a reed), a writing pen.

cal'culus, i (dim. of *calx,* a lump of lime), a pebble, a stone

capil'lus, i (cf. *caput,* the head), a hair of the head.

carpus, i (fr. *carpo,* to pluck), the wrist.

caryophyl'lus, i (κάρυον, walnut; φύλλον, leaf), clove tree.

clavus, i (cf. *clavis,* a bolt or key), a nail; a corn; sick headache.

con'gius, i (cognate with κόγχη, a shell), a gallon.

morbus, i (allied to *morior,* to die), a disease.

natu'ra, æ (fr. *nascor,* to be born), that which will produce, nature.

neb'ula, æ (dim. of *nubes,* a cloud), a haze.

nympha, æ (Greek νυμφή, a nymph or bride), a nymph; *labium minus.*

ret'ina, æ (fr. *rete,* a net), belonging to a net; retina.

offici'na, æ (fr. *opifex,* doing work), a work-shop, drug-store.

oleoresi'na, æ (*oleum,* oil; *resina,* resin), oleo-resin.

or'bita, æ (fr. *orbis,* a circle, orb), the orbit, eye-socket.

in, in.   **a, ab,** from.

A. 1. Bacilli morbi. 2. Acini glandulae. 3. Fistula in ano. 4. Sunt alveoli in maxilla. 5. Folia caryophylli. 6. Congius aquae menthae. 7. Nebula corneae. 8. In officina sunt oleo-resinae et misturae. 9. Calculi in orbita. 10. Clavus digitorum.

B. In the apothecary shop are mixtures and a gallon of rose water. 2. The sockets of the jaw-bones. 3. A ball of arrow-root. 4. Sick headache is a disease. 5. In the orbit there are an artery and a network. 6. The little ring of the cornea. 7. In the retina are small rods. 8. The membrane of the nipple. 9. In the breast are kernels (acini). 10. A pound of cloves.

There are a few nouns of the second declension ending in *er*. *Cancer* (cognate with χάρχινος, a crab) a crab, or cancer, is declined as follows: —

	SINGULAR.	PLURAL.
Nom.	canc er, a cancer	canc ri, cancers
Gen.	canc ri	canc ro'rum
Dat.	canc ro	canc ris
Acc.	canc rum	canc ros
Voc.	canc er	canc ri
Abl.	canc ro	canc ris

VOCABULARY IV.

liber, bri, the bark of a tree; a book; cf. A. S. *boc,* beach.

puer, pu'eri (cf. Greek παῖς, a boy) a boy.

puel'la æ (dim. fem. of *puer*) a girl.

vir, viri (cf. *vis,* strength) a male; man.

pupil'la, æ (dim. of *pupa,* a doll) the pupil.

palma, æ (Greek παλάμη, palm) palm of hand or sole.

patel'la, æ (dim. of *patina,* a pan) the knee-pan.

phytolac'ca, æ (Greek φύτον, plant, and λάκκος, pond) poke plant.

pil'ula, æ (dim. of *pila,* a ball) a little ball ; a pill.

planta, æ (cognate with πλατύς, flat) a plant; the sole of the foot.

porta, æ (cf. *porto,* to carry) the place through which things are carried; a gate.

ran'ula, æ (dim. of *rana,* a frog) tumor of salivary gland.

resi'na, æ (cf. ρητίνα, a gum) resin.

rose'ola, æ (dim. of *rosa,* a rose) rose rash.

rube'ola, æ (dim. of *ruber,* red) measles.

fascic'ulus, i (dim. of *fascis,* a bundle) a little bundle.

focus, i (fr. an old root, *fo;* cf. *foveo,* to boil) a fire-place.

fundus, i (*fundo,* to found) the bottom; lowest port.

funic'ulus, i (dim. of *funis,* a rope) a string; umbilical cord.

gladi'olus, i (dim. of *gladius,* a sword) a part of sternum.

globus, i (like *glomus,* a ball) a ball ; a globe.

cer'ebrum, i (cf. κάρα, the head) the greater brain.

habet, has.　　　　**habent,** have.

EXERCISE IV.

A. 1. Pilulae aloes et mastiches. 2. Plantae pueri et viri. 3. Cancer mammae est morbus feminarum. 4. Rubeola et roseola morbi sunt. 5. Quinina medicina anginae est. 6. Liber medici est in officina. 7. Eucalyptus est malariae medicina. 8. Libra foliorum phytolaccae. 9. Femina neuralgiam orbitae habet. 10. Viri gladiolos habent.

B. 1. A little bundle of small rods. 2. Cancer of the brain is a disease. 3. The physician (medicus) has pills of aloes and myrrh. 4. The boys and girls have measles. 5. The books of the men are in the office. 6. Pepsin is a medicine for dyspepsia. 7. In the *conjunctiva* is the gate of tears. 8. Ranula in the cheek (*mala*) of the girl. 9. Rose rash is a disease. 10. The woman has the hysterical (*hystericum*) globe.

8

GREEK NOUNS OF THE SECOND DECLENSION.

A few nouns of Greek origin ending in *os* are found in medical works, used only in the singular The word *asbes'tos*, from *ἀ*, intensive, *σβέννυμι*, to quench, because it will not burn, is declined as follows :—

Nom.	**asbes'tos**
Gen.	**asbes'ti**
Dat.	**asbes'to**
Acc.	**asbes'ton**
Voc.	**asbes'te**
Abl.	**asbes'to**

A much larger number end in *on*, such as those derived from *φυτόν* (*phyton*), a plant, *ζῶον* (*zoon*), an animal, *δένδρον* (*dendron*), a tree, and *σπόρον* (*sporon*), a spore.

Ganglion (Greek *γάγγλιον*, a knot, a tumor) is thus declined :—

	SINGULAR.	PLURAL.
Nom.	**gang'lion**	**gang'lia**
Gen.	**gang'lii**	**ganglio'rum**
Dat.	**gang'lio**	**gang'liis**
Acc.	**gang'lion**	**gang'lia**
Voc.	**gang'lion**	**gang'lia**
Abl.	**gang'lio**	**gang'liis**

VOCABULARY V.

am'nion, or **am'nios,** i (fr. Greek *ἀμνός*, a lamb, from its softness) a fœtal membrane.

cho'rion, i (Greek *χορίον*, leather) a tough fœtal membrane.

epip'loon, i (Greek *ἐπί*, upon, *πλέω*, to fold) omentum.

hæmatox'ylon, i (Greek *αἷμα*, blood, and *ξύλον*, wood) logwood.

hydrozo'on, i (Greek *ὕδωρ*, water, *ζῶον*, animal) water animalcule.

lirioden'dron, i (Greek λείριον, a lily, δένδρον, tree) tulip tree.

olec'ranon, i (Greek ὠλένη, elbow, and κράνον, head) head of ulna.

pleuron, i (Greek πλεῦρον, the side) the serous covering of the lungs.

micros'poron, i (Greek μικρός, small, σπορός, a spore) a microscopic spore.

sali'va, æ (cf Greek σίαλον, spittle) spittle.

scap'ula, æ (cf. Greek σκάφος, skiff) shoulder blade.

scarlati'na, æ (fr. Italian *scarlatto*, scarlet) scarlet fever.

scilla, æ (Greek σκίλλα, an onion) squill.

serpenta'ria, æ (fr. *serpo*, to creep) Virginia snake-root.

scutella'ria, æ (dim. of *scutum*, a shield) skull cap.

spige'lia, æ (fr. Spigelius, the Dutch anatomist) pink root.

spina, æ (contraction of *spicna*, a point) a thorn, spine.

stria, æ (fr. *strio*, to groove) a groove, colored line.

sutu'ra, æ (fr. *suo*, to sew) a seam, suture.

hu'mulus, i (fr. *humus*, the ground) hop plant.

lob'ulus, i (dim. of *lobus*, a lobe) a small lobe, lobule.

locus, i (originally *stlocus*, cogn. w. στέλλω, to send) a place.

mal'leus, i (cf. Sansk. *mah*, to strike) a hammer; a bone of the ear.

malle'olus, i (dim. of *malleus*) a small hammer, ankle tuberosities.

mus'culus, i (dim. of *mus*, a mouse, or Greek μῦς, a muscle) a muscle.

nævus, i (contraction of *nativus*, fr. *nascor*, to be born) a birth-mark.

nanus, i (Greek νᾶνος, a pigmy) a dwarf.

nervus, i (fr. same root as νεῦρον) a nerve.

nodus, i (fr. *gnodus*, a knot) a knot, node.

nu'cleus, i (dim. of *nux*, a nut) a kernel.

nucle'olus, i (dim. of *nucleus*) primary nucleus.

pilocar'pus, i (*pila,* ball, *carpus,* fruit) jaborandi.

ruga, æ (fr. Aryan root *rag,* rough) a wrinkle.

ruta, æ Greek ρυτή, rue) rue.

sabba'tia, æ (fr. Sabbati, an Italian botanist) sabbatia.

sabi'na, æ (fr. a town in ancient Italy; a Sabine woman) savine.

salici'na, æ (fr. *salix,* a willow) alkaloid from willow.

sanguina'ria, æ (fr. *sanguis,* blood, from color of juice) bloodroot.

sen'ega, æ (fr. Indian *Seneka*) corrupted into *snake* root.

sil'ica, æ (fr. *silex,* flint) oxide of silicon.

non, not.

EXERCISE V.

A. 1. Musculi strias habent.   2. Scapula fossam habet.   3. Scrofula est morbus puerorum.   4. Corona spinarum.   5. Nervi ganglia habent.   6. Scilla medicina morbis est pleuri.   7. Amnion et chorion sunt membranae. Icterus et scarlatina morbi sunt.   9. Cerebrum lobos habet.   10. Hydrozoa non plantae sunt.

B. 1. The physician gives pills of salicin to the boy.   2. Nerves have ganglia but not furrows.   3. Men have muscles, nerves, and arteries.   4. Chalk mixture is a medicine for diarrhœa.   5. Pills of sanguinaria and and ammonia for disease of the pleura.   6. Silica is not a medicine.   7. The women have savine and ergot. 8. Glands have nuclei.   9. The nodes of the nerves. 10. The dwarf has a birth-mark.

CHAPTER VII.

The Third Declension.

NOUNS of the third declension have various endings in the nominative singular but the genitive singular always ends in *is;* sometimes with an increment (*i. e.* additional syllable) and *is*, sometimes by the addition of *is* to the nominative singular, and sometimes, when the nominative singular ends in *is*, the word is not changed in the genitive. *Metus*, fear, for example, forms the genitive singular *metoris;* the *or* being the increment and *is* the termination. *Tremor*, trembling, simply adds *is*, while *classis*, a class or fleet, remains unchanged.

The student must commit to memory the termination of the genitive singular and the gender of all words of this declension.

Arbor, a tree, is declined as follows:—

	SINGULAR.	PLURAL.
Nom.	arbor (m)	arb'ores
Gen.	arb'oris	arb'orum
Dat.	arb'ori	arbor'ibus
Acc.	arb'orem	arb'ores
Voc.	arbor	arb'ores
Abl.	arb'ore	arbor'ibus

Nouns of the third declension ending in *or* are usually of the masculine gender. The words in the following vocabulary are declined like *arbor*.

VOCABULARY VI.

abduc′tor, o′ris (m) (from *ab*, away, *duco*, to lead) an abductor.

aer, a′eris (m) (Greek ἀήρ, air) air.

anser, an′seris (m) (allied to *ansa*, a handle, fr. long neck) a goose.

æther, æth′eris (Greek αἰθήρ, ether) ether.

ardor, o′ris (*ardeo*, to burn with zeal) a burning.

calor, o′ris (*calco*, to be warm) heat.

climac′ter, e′ris (Greek κλιμακτήρ, a round of a ladder) a critical period.

croton, o′nis (Gk. κροτών, dog tick) palma Christi plant.

dila′tor, o′ris (*dis*, apart, *fero*, to bear) dilator.

erec′tor, o′ris (fr. *erigo*, to stand up) erector.

exten′sor, o′ris (*ex*, out, and *tendo*, to stretch) extensor.

flexor, o′ris (*fligo*, to bend) bender.

fluor, o′ris (*fluo*, to flow) a flowing.

furfur, fur′furis (reduplication of *far*, a cereal) bran.

humor, o′ris (cf. χυμός, a liquid) a moisture, humor.

labor, o′ris (cf. *labor*, to slip) labor, parturition.

leva′tor o′ris (fr. *levo*, to lift) a lifter.

lichen, e′nis (Greek λειχήν), a cryptogamous plant.

limon, o′nis (from Portuguese town Limoa or Persian *limun*) lemon.

liquor, o′ris (fr. *liquco*, to be fluid) fluidity; liquid, solution.

motor, o′ris (fr. *moveo*, to move) mover.

prona′tor, o′ris (from *prono*, to bend forward) a bender forward.

ren, is (cf. φρήν, the diaphragm) the reins, kidneys.

rigor, o′ris (fr. *rigeo*, to be numb) a chill.

rota′tor, o′ris (fr. *roto*, to turn) roller.

rubor, o′ris (fr. *rubus*, red) redness, blushing.

sal, is (cf. Greek ἅλς, salt) salt.

sopor, o′ris (cf. Greek ὀπός, juice) sleep.

sphincter, e′ris (Greek σφίγγω, to squeeze) contractor.
stertor, o′ris (onomatopœic) snoring.
stupor, o′ris (fr. *stupeo;* cf. τύπτω, to strike senseless)
    insensibility.
sudor, o′ris (fr. *sudo,* to sweat; cf. ὕδωρ, water) sweat.
tumor, o′ris (fr. *tumeo,* to swell) a tumor, swelling.
trochan′ter, e′ris (Greek τροχόω. to roll) a roller; process
tensor, o′ris (fr. *tendo,* to stretch) a stretcher.
vapor, o′ris (cognate with κάπνος, smoke) smoke, steam,

    aliquando, sometimes.
    dat, gives.   **dant,** give.

EXERCISE VI.

A. 1. Feminae aliquando anseres sunt. 2. Vir nervos motores habet. 3. Flexores et extensores humeri. 4. Anus levatorem et sphincteres habet. 5. Sunt aliquando in morbis rigores et calor. 6. Fluor humorum est causa morborum. 7. Motores carpi musculi. 8. Microsporon furfur planta est. 9. Renes viri lobos habent. 10. Aliquando in morbis sunt stertor, sudor, stupor, tremor, et sopor.

B. 1. Vapor of water and salt of ammonia. 2. The trembling, snoring and sluggishness of disease. 3. The liquids of ammonia and potash (potassa). 4. The fluid of the amnion. 5. Women have critical periods. 6. The lifters of the ribs. 7. The sweat and tears of the women. 8. Ether is not air. 9. The stretchers and benders of the carpus. 10. The physician gives a drachm of jalap to the man.

Some neuter nouns of the third declension form the genitive like the above by adding *is* to the nominative. The accusative and vocative cases in both numbers are like the nominative.

Sometimes a final *l* or *s* of the nominative is doubled when the termination of an oblique case is added.   *Vas* (from same root as Sanskrit *vasti*, a bladder, and Latin *vesica*) is declined as follows:—

	SINGULAR.	PLURAL.
Nom.	vas. a vessel	vasa, vessels
Gen.	vasis	vasum
Dat.	vasi	vas'ibus
Acc.	vas	vasa
Voc.	vas	vasa
Abl.	vase	vas'ibus

VOCABULARY VII.

an'imal, ā'lis (n) (fr. *anima*, vital principle) animal.

cada'ver, ĕris (n) (fr. *cado*, to fall in battle) a corpse.

fel, fellis (n) (kindred with *bilis*, bile) bile, gall.

mel, mellis (n) (Greek μέλι, whence, μέλισσα, a bee) honey.

os, ossis (n) (cf. Sanskrit *osthi*, a bone) a bone.

pulmo, ōnis (fr. πλεύμων, for πνεύμων) the lung.

stear, is (n) (Greek στέαρ, tallow) stiff grease, tallow.

tuber, eris (n) (for *timber* from *tumeo*) a bulb.

tab'ula, æ (fr. the root *tab*, flat surface) a table.

tae'nia, æ (Greek ταινία, from τείνω to stretch) a tape, ribbon; tape-worm.

terebin'thina, æ (fr. Gk. τερεβίνθος, pine tree) turpentine.

terra, æ (kindred with *torreo*, to dry) earth.

testa, æ (allied to *tosta*, parched) a shell.

tib'ia, æ (cf. *tabeo*, to waste away) a flute, shin-bone.

tinctu'ra, æ (fr. *tingo*, to dye) a tincture.

tin'ea, æ (perhaps from τίνω, to punish) a bookworm; ringworm.

tu'nica, æ, a close-fitting undergarment, tunic, covering.

octa'rius, i (fr. *octo*, eight) the eighth of a *congius;* a pint.

oc'ulus, i (dim.; cf. Ionic ὄκκος) an eye.

pedic'ulus, i (dim. of *pes*, a foot) a small foot; pedicle; a louse.

papy'rus, i (Greek πάπυρος, the paper-reed) parchment.

ace'tum, i (fr. past part. of *acco,* to become sour) sour
   wine; vinegar.

curat, cures.   **curant,** cure.

EXERCISE VII.

A.   1. Mistura fellis et mellis.   2. Ossa tubera et
pediculos habent.   3. Chirurgus (surgeon) cancros et
tumores curat   4. Medicus rubeolam et scarlatinam
curat.   5. Animalia ossa et musculos habent.   6. Octarius tincturae zingiberis.   7. Arteriae vasa vaso*r*um (fr.
vasum, a vessel) habent.   8. Medicus curat tineam cum
terebenthina.   9. Tabulae et laminae ossium.   10. Drachma aceti scillae.

B.   1. The shell of the earth.   2. The covering of
the eyes.   3. The physician gives vinegar to the boy.
4. Tinctures of rhubarb and ammonia.   5. There is gall
in the vessel.   6. The corpse is on the table.   7. The
shin-bone has lines and grooves.   8. A pint of tincture
of squill.   9. There is paper in the book.   10. The animal has bones, tallow, and nerves.

Many nouns of the third declension ending in *is* in
the nominative singular remain unchanged in the genitive.

   Avis (f), a bird (allied to Greek ἄω, to move the
air), is declined as follows:—

	SINGULAR.	PLURAL.
Nom.	avis, a bird	aves, birds
Gen.	avis, of a bird	a'vium, of birds
Dat.	avi	av'ibus
Acc.	avem	aves
Voc.	avis	aves
Abl.	ave, or i	av'ibus

All the nouns of the third declension in the following vocabulary are similarly declined.

VOCABULARY VIII.

apis (f) (fr. *apo*, to fasten) the clinging animal; a bee.

auris (f) (fr. same root as Greek οὖς, the ear) an ear.

axis (m) (Greek ἀξών, an axle, fr. ἄγω, to carry) an axle-tree; second vertebra.

basis (f) (Greek βάσις, a pedestal) foundation, base.

crinis (m) (fr. *cer*, as seen in *cresco*, to grow) the hair.

cutis (f) (kindred to κύτος, a bag of leather) the skin.

digita'lis (f) (fr. *digitus*, a finger, or *digitale*, a glove finger) foxglove.

febris (f) (fr. *ferbis* fr. *ferveo*, to be warm) a fever.

funis (m) (fr. a root meaning to bind) a rope, cord.

ignis (m) (Sanskrit *agnis*) fire.

naris (f) (cf. πνέω, to breathe, *nasum*, the nose) a nostril.

panis (m) (perhaps fr. *Pan*, a demigod of the fields) bread.

pelvis (f) (allied to Greek πύελος, basin) basin, pelvis.

pertus'sis (f) (fr. *per* intens. and *tussis*, cough) whooping cough.

piscis (m) (perhaps allied to *pascor*, feed upon) a fish.

sina'pis (f) (Greek σίναπυ, mustard) mustard.

sitis (f) (*sitio*, to be dry) thirst.

taxis (f) (from Greek τάσσω, to draw) reduction by handling.

testis (m) (fr. *testa*, a shell, because witnesses voted with shells in determining the guilt of the accused) a witness; evidence; testicle.

vis, acc. *vim*, pl. *vires* (cf. Gk. ἵς, fibre) strength, power.

ulna, æ (fr. Gk. ὠλένη, the elbow) ulna; elbow bone.

un'cia, æ (Greek οὐγκία, 1-12 of a pound) an ounce.

urtica'ria, æ (from *urtica*, a nettle, fr. *uro*, to burn) nettle rash.

uva, æ (kindred to *uveo*, to be moist) a grape.

u'vula, æ (dim. of *uva*, a grape) small grape; uvula.

causat, causes.   **causant**, cause.

EXERCISE VIII.

A. 1. Axis et ulna ossa sunt. 2. In febribus sunt crises et lyses. 3. Tinea et urticaria sunt morbi cutis. 4. Feminae pelves habent. 6. Terebenthina ardorem urinae causat. 6. Octarius aceti et drachma tincturae digitalis. 7. Calor, aer, et aqua sunt medicinae. 8. Ipecacuanha et digitalis fluorem urinae causant. 9. Puer pisces et panem habet. 10. Puella pertussem habet.

B. 1. The wings of the birds. 2. The nostrils have dilators and depressors. 3. A pint of vinegar and water for the thirst of fever. 4. An ounce of tincture of foxglove. 5. Gonorrhœa causes a burning of the urine. 6. Bees have antennae but not ears. 7. The surgeon cures the tumor with fire. 8. A crumb of bread. 9. The woman has fish and mustard in the basin. 10. The power of nature is a physician.

Nouns of the third declension ending in *men*, a termination originally added to the root of verbs to form nouns denoting the result of the verbal action, are of the neuter gender. They form the genitive singular by changing the *e* of the final syllable to *i* and adding the genitive termination *is*. *Cerumen*, ear wax, (from *cera*, bleached wax), is thus declined:—

	SINGULAR.	PLURAL.
Nom.	ceru′men	ceru′mina
Gen.	ceru′minis	ceru′minum
Dat.	ceru′mini	cerumin′ibus
Acc.	ceru′men	ceru′mina
Voc.	ceru′men	ceru′mina
Abl.	ceru′mine	cerumin′ibus

VOCABULARY IX.

abdo'men, inis (fr. *abdo*, to hide) the belly.
albu'men, inis (fr. *albus*, white) white of egg; albumen.
alu'men, inis (allied to ἅλς, salt) alum.
cacu'men, inis (fr. *acumen*, a point, with prefix *c*) top of a plant.
fora'men, inis (fr. *foro*, to bore) a hole, orifice.
gramen, inis (alteration of *cremen*, growth) grass.
inguen, inis (fr. *inquino*, to befoul) the groin.
moli'men, inis (fr. *molior*, to struggle) a bearing down pain.
pecten, inis (Gk. πεκτήν, a comb) comb; os pubis.
semen, inis (fr. *sero*, to sow) seed.
stamen, inis (from *sto*, to stand) a standard; stamen of flower.
tormen, inis (from *torqueo*, to twist) a writhing, twisting pain.
vagi'na, æ (kindred with φάγω, to swallow) a sheath, vagina.
valva, æ (fr. *volvo*, to turn) a folding door, valve.
vulva, æ (altered fr. *volva*, fr. *volvco*, to wrap) a wrapper; vulva.
vari'ola, æ (dim. of *varus*, a blotch) small-pox.
varicel'la, æ (dim. of *varix*, a pimple) chicken pox.
vena, æ (possibly allied to φαίνω, to be evident because on surface) a vein.
vesi'ca, æ cf. *vas*, a vessel) a bladder.
via, æ (fr. *ire*, to go) a way, track.
vi'ola, æ (Greek ἴον, a violet) a violet.
vita, æ (fr. *vivo*, to live) life.
zona, æ (Greek ζωνή, a belt) a belt, girdle, zone.

EXERCISE IX.

A. 1. Renes in abdomine sunt. 2. Cacumen violae. Sphincter vaginae. 3. In tibia sunt foramina. 4. Vena

portae in abdomine est.   5. Vir cerumen in auribus
habet.   6. Tinctura valerianae est hysteriae medicina.
6. Venae et calculus vesicae.   8. Habet albumen in
urina.   9. Feminae molimina et tormina habent.   10. Puer
gramen animalibus dat.

 B.   1. Alum is a medicine for diseases of the nose.
2. The veins and arteries of bones.   3. In diseases of the
kidneys there is albumen in the urine.   4. Life is a road
of thorns.   5. The accelerator of the urine is the ejacu-
lator of the seed.   6. Twisting pains in the belly.   7. The
bladder has a squeezing muscle.   8. In the fluid of the
amnion there is albumen and salt.   9. The "comb" is
the bone of the pubes.   10. The boy gives grass to the
cows (*vacca*).

Nouns of the third declension ending in *es* usually
change *es* to *is* in forming the genitive singular; thus,
pubes, the pubic hair, genitive *pubis*, of the pubic hair.

 The majority of these words, however, form the
genitive by adding *is* with an increment.

 Caput (neuter), the head (from same root as Greek
χεφαλή and German *kopf*), is declined as follows:—

	SINGULAR.	PLURAL.
Nom.	ca′put, a head	cap′ita, heads
Gen.	cap′itis	cap′itum
Dat.	cap′iti	capit′ibus
Acc.	ca′put	cap′ita
Voc.	ca′put	cap′ita
Abl.	cap′ite	capit′ibus

VOCABULARY X.

ace′tas, a′tis (m) (fr. *acetum*, vinegar) an acetate.
adeps, ad′ipis (m) (fr. Greek *a*, *un*, and root ὀαπ, to tear)
 . lard; stiff grease.

æs, æ'ris (n) (probably fr. *αἶς,* a copper coin) brass.

ætas, a'tis (f) (fr. *ævitas,* fr. *ævum,* an age) age.

albu go, albu'ginis (f) (fr. *albus,* white) white of eye.

anthrax, a'cis (m) (Gk. *ἄνθραξ,* burning coal) carbuncle.

apex, ap'icis (m) (possibly fr. *apo,* to fasten) a point, top.

appen dix, appen'dicis (f) (fr. *ad,* to, and *pendeo.* to hang) appendix.

atlas, atlan'tis (m) (Gk. *Ἄτλας,* the god who supported the world on his shoulders) the first vertebra.

cory za, æ (fr. Gk. *κάρα,* head, and *ζέω,* to boil) cold in the head.

pilus, i, a hair.

pinus, i (f) (kindred to Greek *πίτυς,* pine) a pine tree.

prunus, i (f) (Greek *προύνη,* a plum tree) wild cherry.

porus, i (Gk. *πόρος,* a passage) a pore.

pyrus, i (f) (fr. the country *Epirus*) a pear tree.

absin thium, i (fr. *Ἀψίνθιοι,* a people in Southern Thrace) wormwood.

ac idum, i (fr. *aceo,* to be sour) an acid.

al lium, i (probably fr. *alius,* because imported) a garlic.

ammoni acum, i (fr. Egyptian through Greek *Ἄμμων,* the tree growing near the temple of Jupiter Ammon) ammoniac.

am'ylum, i (*ἀ, un,* and *μύλη,* mill, not ground) starch.

animal'culum,* i (dim. of *animal*) microscopic animal.

ani'sum, i (fr. Greek *ἀνίημι,* to send up an odor) anise.

ver tebra, æ (*verto,* to turn) a spindle; a vertebra.

EXERCISE X.

A. 1. Libra adipis et uncia ammonii acetatis. 2. Anthrax est morbus animalium. 3. Apices pulmonum. 4. Pori cutis et pili capitis. 5. Atlas et axis ver-

---

* *Animalcula* is the plural of *animalculum.* There is no such word as *animalculæ.*

tebrae sunt. 6. Pinus et prunus sunt arbores. 7. Urticaria est morbus cutis et nervorum. 8. Medicus guttam tincturae aconiti puero dat. 9. Amylum et albumen cibus (food) virorum sunt. 10. In aqua sunt animalcula et plantae.

B. 1. Tincture of aconite is a medicine for fevers. 2. Animalcules in vinegar. 3. The atlas is not a bone of the head. 4. Lard and starch are foods. 5. Carbuncle is a skin disease. 6. The age of brass.

GREEK NOUNS OF THE THIRD DECLENSION.

There are many Greek nouns of the third declension, all of which originally formed the genitive singular in *os*. The majority of these words end in *is*, as *diuresis*, *catharsis*.

Catharsis, purging, from *κατά*, down, *αἴρω*, to take, and *calomelas* calomel are thus declined:—

	SINGULAR.	SINGULAR.
Nom.	cathar′sis	calom′elas
Gen.	cathar′seos	calomel′anos
Dat.	cathar′si	calomel′ani
Acc.	cathar′sin	calomel′ana
Voc.	cathar′sis	calom′elas
Abl.	cathar′si	calomel′ane

Pure Greek words like the above are not found in the plural in medical works. Of late there is a tendency to employ the regular Latin terminations of the third declension, but there is no good reason for so doing.

Another large class of Greek words end in *tis* and *ma*. These originally made the genitive singular in *idos* and *atos*, but now *idis* and *atis* are preferred; thus, *bronchitis* forms the genitive *bronchitidis*, and *exanthema*, *exanthematis*. Those ending in *tis* are feminine; those ending in *ma* are neuter.

Rhus (fem.), sumac, ivy (from Greek ῥοῦς, gen. ῥοός) and *aletris*, are declined as follows:—

SINGULAR.	SINGULAR.
Nom. rhus, ivy	al'etris (f), star grass
Gen. rhois	alet'ridis
Dat. rhoi	alet'ridi
Acc. rhoem or en	alet'ridem or en
Voc. rhus	al'etris
Abl. rhoe or i	alet'ride

Words like the above are used only in the singular. The nouns of this declension ending in *ma* are used in both numbers.

Enema, a clyster, from ἐνίημι, to inject, is thus declined:—

SINGULAR.	PLURAL.
Nom. en'ema, clyster	enem'ata, clysters
Gen. enem'atis	enem'atum
Dat. enem'ati	enemat'ibus
Acc. en'ema	enem'ata
Voc. en'ema	enem'ata
Abl. enem'ati or e	enemat'ibus

VOCABULARY XI.

al'etris, idis (f) (Gk. ἀλετρίς, a female slave who grinds corn) star grass.

am'yris, idis (f) (Gk. ἀ, intensive, and μύρον, odorous juice) amyris.

aphis, idis (f) (Greek ἀφίς, a louse) a plant louse.

arthri'tis, idis (f) (Greek ἀρθρῖτις) inflammation of a joint.

as'caris, idis (f) (Gk. ἀσκαρίς, a maw worm) pin-worm.

asclep'ias, adis (f) (fr. Ἀσκλέπιας, Æsculapius) milkweed.

colocyn'this, idis (f) (fr. κολοκύνθη, pumpkin) colocynth.

hamame'lis, idis (f) (from ἅμα, like, and μῆλον, an apple) witch hazel.

119

coma, atis (n) (Greek κῶμα, deep sleep) coma.

glottis, idis (f) (fr. γλῶττα, the tongue) the glottis.

gramma, atis (n) (Gk. γράμμα, a letter, a coin) a gram.

hepar, atis (n) (Greek ἧπαρ, liver) liver.

hydras'tis, idis (f) (fr. ὕδωρ, water) golden seal.

juglans, ndis (f) (*Jovis*, of Jove, *glans*, nut) butternut.

lapis, idis (f) (cf. Greek λᾶας, a stone) a stone.

mias'ma, atis (n) (fr. Greek μιάζω, to contaminate) an effluvium.

physostig'ma, atis (n) (from Greek φύσις, growth, στίγμα head) Calabar bean.

phosphis, i'tis (m) (fr. φῶς, light) a phosphite.

plasma, atis (n) (fr. Greek πλάσσω, to form) plasma.

pneuma, atis (n) (fr. Gk. πνεῦμα) a gaseous substance.

pyr'amis, idis (f) (possibly fr. πῦρ, fire) a pyramid.

rheuma, atis (n) (fr. Gk. ῥέω, to flow) a humor.

rhizo'ma, atis (n) (fr. Gk. ῥίζα, a root) root stock.

stigma, atis (n) (fr. Gk. στίζω, to point) the top of a pistil.

sulphis, i'tis (m) (sulphur) a sulphite.

sympto'ma, atis (n) (σύν, together, πίπτω, to fall) symptom

syste'ma, atis (n) (σύν. together, ἵστημι, to stand) system.

theobro'ma, atis (n) (θεός, god, βρῶμα, food) cocoa.

antrum, i (Greek ἄντρον, a cave) a cavity.

arca'num, i (fr. *arcco*, to shut up) a nostrum.

EXERCISE XI.

A.   1. Rubor et tumor symptomata arthritidis sunt. 2. Medicus enema hydrastidis puero dat.   3. Morbus oculorum symptoma syphilidis est.   4. Gramma sodii phosphitis et uncia theobromatis.   5. Hepar sulphuris morbis cutis.   6. Fel in urina est symptoma morbi hepatis.   7. Pyramides renum.   8. Miasmata causae februm sunt.   9. In corpore sunt arcana naturae.   10. In exanthematibus sunt maculae, papulae, et bullae.

9

B.   1. An ounce of tincture of golden seal.   2. A pound of star grass in a gallon of water.   3. In the cavity of the jaw-bone there is a membrane.   4. A pint of tincture of agave in the shop.   5. The man has cancer of the liver and kidneys.   6. In the bladder there are sometimes pebbles, but not stones.   7. The rootstock of ivy is not a medicine.   8. A gramme of sulphite of soda in water.   9. The nerves, veins, and lobes of the liver.   10. Macules and papules are symptoms of syphilis.

CHAPTER VIII.

The Fourth Declension.

NOUNS of the fourth declension form the genitive singular in *us*, the *u* being a contraction of the earlier ending *uis*, and is, therefore, long in quantity; e. g., *manus*, a hand, genitive *manus*, of a hand. The *us* of the genitive is sometimes written with the circumflex accent in order to distinguish it from the nominative singular.

Nouns of this declension ending in *us* are masculine with the exception of *manus*, a hand, *acus*, a needle, and the names of plants, which are feminine.

Nouns of the fourth declension ending in *u* are of the neuter gender.

The genitive plural ends in *uum*, the dative plural in *ibus*, except *acus*, a needle, *arcus*, a bow, *artus*, a joint, *lacus*, a lake, and *partus*, a birth, which form the dative plural in *ubus*.

Manus (fem.) a hand (fr. Aryan root *ma*, to measure) is declined as follows:—

	SINGULAR.	PLURAL.
Nom.	manus, a hand	manus, hands
Gen.	manus	man'uum
Dat.	man'ui	man'ibus
Acc.	manum	manus
Voc.	manus	manus
Abl.	manu	man'ibus

VOCABULARY XII.

abor'tus, ûs (*aborior*, to rise from a losing game) abortion.
absces'sus, ûs (*abs*, from, and *cedo*, go) departure, abscess.
afflux'us, ûs (*ad*, to, and *fluo*, to flow) a flowing to, afflux.

appara′tus, ûs (*ad*, for, *paratus*, ready) instruments, apparatus.

aqueduc′tus, ûs (*aqua*, water, *ductus*, a duct) a water way, aqueduct.

audi′tus, ûs (fr. *audio*, to hear) hearing.

co′itus, ûs (*cum*, together, *irc*, to go) intercourse (sexual).

congres′sus, ûs (*cum*, together, *gradior*, to walk) coitus.

cornus, ûs (f) (fr. *cornu*, a horn, on account of its hard wood) dogwood.

cu′bitus, ûs (fr. *cubo*, to lie down) lying down.

decu′bitus, ûs (*dc*, from, *cubitus*, lying) position in lying.

ductus, ûs (fr. *duco*, to lead) a duct.

flatus, ûs (fr. *flo*, to blow) gas in bowels.

fluxus, ûs (fr. *fluo*, to flow) a flowing; flux.

fœtus, ûs (fr. *fco*, to produce) unborn child.

fructus, ûs (fr. *fruor*, to enjoy) that which is enjoyed; fruit.

gustus, ûs (fr. *gusto*, to taste) that which tastes; sense of taste.

hab′itus, ûs (fr. *habco*, to have or acquire) habit.

hal′itus, ûs (fr. *halo*, to breathe) breath, vapor.

haustus, ûs (fr. *haurio*, to drink) a draught.

ictus, ûs (fr. *ico*, to smite) a stroke.

lusus, ûs (fr. *ludo*, to play) a sport, joke.

motus, ûs (fr. *moveo*, to move) motion.

nisus, ûs (fr. *nitor*, to struggle, bear down) an effort; bearing down.

olfac′tus, ûs (fr. *olco*, to emit an odor, and *facio*, to make) sense of smell.

ra′dius, i (cf. ῥίζα, a root) a staff; a spoke; the radius.

ramus, i (kindred with *radix*, a root) a branch.

ranun′culus, i (f) (dim. of *rana*, a frog) crowfoot.

rhamnus, i (f) (Greek ῥάμνος, buckthorn) buckthorn.

ric′inus, i (f) (fr. root *phric*, to rub) castor oil plant.

tor′cular, is (n) (fr. *torqueo*, to twist) a wine-press.

EXERCISE XII.

A. 1. Medicus abortum curat. 2. Animal abscessum hepatis habet. 3. Aqueductus Sylvii et cochleae. 4. In decubitu peritonitidis. 5. Inflammatio artuum manus. 6. Ictus solis est morbus systematis nervorum. 7. Monstrositates sunt lusus naturae. 8. Pronatores radii. 9. Venae et ductus fœtus. 10. Fœtus nisum feminae causat.

B. 1. A draught of tincture of valerian. 2. The branches and buds of the trees. 3. The bones of the head and the joints of the hands. 4. The surgeon has needles and apparatus. 5. The man has sunstroke. 6. The nerves of smell, hearing and taste. 7. Crowfoot and buckthorn are plants. 8. The bodies, arches, and pedicles of the vertebrae. 9. The position of the body in inflammation of the joints. 10. A bad (*mala*) mixture of the humors is the cause of disease, says (*ait*) Galen.

———————

It will be observed that the great majority of nouns of the fourth declension ending in *us* are of verbal origin, being derived from the supine or past participle. They denote the action expressed by the verb; thus, *audio*, to hear, *auditus*, hearing; *sentio*, to feel or *sense* a thing, *sensus*, sensation; *volo*, to will or wish, *vultus*, that which expresses the will and desires, *i. e.*, the countenance.

There are but few neuter nouns of this declension. They are all very ancient, being found in the oldest specimens of Latin. It is quite probable that many nouns originally belonging to the fourth declension were converted into nouns of the second or third declensions.

Cornu, a horn (kindred with κέρας and German *horn*) is declined as follows:—

SINGULAR.		PLURAL.	
Nom.	cornu, a horn	cor'nua, horns	
Gen.	cornus, of a horn	cor'nuum	
Dat.	cor'nui	cor'nibus	
Acc.	cornu	cor'nua	
Voc.	cornu	cor'nua	
Abl.	cornu	cor'nibus	

VOCABULARY XIII.

genu, ûs (fr. same root as Greek γόνυ, a knee) a knee.

passus, ûs (fr. *pando*, to pace) a pace, step.

plexus, ûs (from *plecto*, to weave) a network of nerves or vessels.

potus, ûs (fr. *poto*, to drink) a drink; drinking.

proces'sus, ûs (from *pro*, forward, and *cedo*, to go) a projection.

prolap'sus, ûs (fr. *pro*, forward, and *labor*, to slip) a slipping forward.

pulsus, ûs (fr. *pello*, to drive) a driving; the pulse.

risus, ûs (fr. *rideo*, to laugh) a laughing, smile.

sexus, ûs (perhaps fr. *seco*, to divide, distinguish) sex.

sinus, ûs (*sinuo*, to swell out like a sail) a fold, bay, gulf, cul-de-sac.

situs, ûs (fr. *sino*, to locate) a location, site.

singul'tus, ûs (from *singuli*, one by one, because of the broken sounds) hiccup, sobbing.

spir'itus, ûs (fr. *spiro*, to breathe) breathing, spirit.

subsul'tus, ûs (from *sub*, up from under, *silio*, to jump) jumping up, twitching.

tactus, ûs (fr. *tango*, to touch) touching, feeling.

tinni'tus, ûs (fr. *tinnio*, to tinkle) tinkling, ringing in ears.

tractus, ûs (fr. *traho*, to draw) a tract, track.

tran'situs, ûs (from *trans*, across, and *ire*, to go) a going
across; transit.

victus, ûs (fr. *vivo*, to live) what one lives on; victuals.

visus, ûs (fr. *video*, to see) seeing; sense of sight.

vom'itus, ûs (fr. *vomo*, to puke) vomiting.

arcus, ûs (anciently *arquus*) a bow, arch.

artus, ûs (fr. ἄρω, to join) a joint.

acus, ûs (f) (fr. *acuo*, to sharpen) a needle.

lacus, ûs (Greek λάκκος, a pond) a lake.

partus, ûs (fr. *pario*, to bring forth) parturition, birth

argen'tum, i (cf. Greek ἀργής, white, shining) silver.

arse'nium, i (fr. ἀρσήν, a male) arsenic.

arum, i (Greek ἄρον, wake-robin) wild turnip.

EXERCISE XIII.

A. 1. Balsamum copaibae est gonorrhœae medicina. 2. Subsultus est symptoma morbi nervorum.
3. Medicus balnea calori febris dat. 4. Quinina tinnitum
aurium causat, aliquando vomitum. 5. Chirurgus sinum
abscessus apparatu curat. 6. In cerebro est plexus vena-
rum, in abdomine plexus nervorum. 7. Viri aliquando
cornua in capite habent. 8. Ossa processus et tubera
habent. 9. Patella artus genus os est. 10. Medicus
potum aquae cum spiritu camphorae puellae dat.

B. 1. The joint of the knee and the bones of the
hand. 2. The man has a slipping forward of the eyes.
3. Abscesses have sinuses and tracts. 4. The site of the
disease is in the liver. 5. The man has hiccup and a
twitching of the muscles. 6. Spirits of æther and ammonia. 7. Salicin and quinine cause ringing of the ears.
8. Diseases of touch, vision, and taste. 9. The man
gives food and drink to the woman. 10. Gold, silver
and barium are metals (*metalla*).

CHAPTER IX.

THE FIFTH DECLENSION.

THERE are a few nouns of the fifth declension used in medical literature. They all end in *es*, and form the genitive singular in *ei*. All nouns of this declension are feminine except *dies*, a day, which is masculine. Only two nouns, *dies*, and *res*, a thing, are declined in all cases, both singular and plural.

Res, a thing (kindred with ῥῆμα, that which is spoken of) is declined as follows:—

	SINGULAR.	PLURAL.
Nom.	res, a thing	res, things
Gen.	rei	rerum
Dat.	rei	rebus
Acc.	rem	res
Voc.	res	res
Abl.	re	rebus

VOCABULARY XIV.

a cies, ē'i (cf. Greek ἀκίς, an edge) an edge.

balbu'ties, ē'i (fr. *balbus*, stammering) stammering.

calvi'ties, ē'i (fr. *calvus*, adj. bald) baldness.

cani'ties, ē'i (fr. *canus*, gray, kindred with κάω, to burn to ashes) ash color; grayness of hair.

ca ries, ē'i (Sanskrit *karkas*, cancer) decay.

fa'cies, ē'i (fr. *facio*, to make) that which is formed; face.

inglu'vies, ē'i (*in*, in, *gula*, gullet) the crop of birds.

ma'cies, ē'i (fr. *macco*, to be lean) leanness, wasting.

molli'ties, ē'i (fr. *mollis*, soft) softening.

ra bies, ē'i (fr. *rabo*, to rave) madness, hydrophobia.

sa nies, ē'i (fr. *sanguis*, blood) blood; fetid matter.

sca'bies, ē'i (fr. *scabo*, to scratch) the itch.

spe'cies, ē'i (fr. *specio*, to look) appearance, variety, look.

spes, ē'i (fr. *spero*, to hope) hope.

superfi cies, ē'i (fr. *super*, upon, and *facies*, the face) upper face; surface.

aspid'ium, i (fr. Gk. ἀσπίδιον, a little shield) shield fern.

aurum, i (old Greek αὖρον, gold, fr. ἄω, to glitter) gold.

bal'neum, i (Greek βαλανεῖον, a bath) a bath.

bal'samum, i (Greek βάλσαμον, fragrant gum) balsam.

ba rium, i (fr. Greek βαρύς, heavy) the metal barium.

benzo'inum, i (from Arabic *benzoah*, a resin from styax) benzoin.

cad'mium, i (fr. καδμεῖα, calamine, fr. *Cadmos*, Thebes, where calamine was first found) cadmium.

EXERCISE XIV.

A. 1. Mollities ossium est morbus puerorum. 2. Ossa faciei et manus. 3. Caries ossium causat fluxum saniei. 4. Rabies est morbus animalium. 5. Febris et phthisis maciem causant. 6. Scabies est species morbi cutis. 7. Canities et calvities symptomata ætatis sunt. 8. Benzoinum est medicina anginae. 9. Calor ictum solis (sun) causat. 10. Aves pennas, alas, et ingluvies habent.

B. 1. He has softening and rottenness of the bones. 2. Grayness and baldness are diseases of the hair. 3. Itch is a disease of boys, rabies of dogs (*canis*). 4. The surface of the bones of the face and head. 5. Tincture of benzoin and oleoresin of sheld fern. 6. The physician has no cadmium in his office. 7. A variety of animalcules causes itch. 8. Hope is nature's medicine. 9. The bloody matter of rotten bone. 10. Stammering and hiccup are diseases of the nerves.

CHAPTER X.

Indeclinable Nouns.

MANY words from languages having no declensions like those of Latin and Greek have been introduced into the pharmacopœias of European countries. These are necessarily used like Latin words, but undergo no changes in the various cases. Indeclinable nouns are all assumed to be of the neuter gender. Thus, we should write *alcohol fortius*, not *alcohol fortior*.

VOCABULARY XV.

buchu, ind. (an African word) buchu.

cat'echu, ind. (a Malay word, *gatchkuah*, boiled juice).

kino, ind. (a word meaning juice) kino.

kousso, ind. (an Abyssinian word) brayera.

sago, ind. (a Malay word, *sagu*, pith) sago.

sas'safras, ind. (a Spanish word, corrupted from Latin *saxifraga*) spleenwort.

rubus, i (f) (fr. *ruber*, red. "*Black*berries are *red* when they are *green*.") a blackberry bush.

saccus, i (Greek σάχχος, a bag) a sac.

scirrhus, i (fr. σχιρρός, hard) a stone cancer.

scopa'rius, i (fr. *scopæ*, twigs for making brooms) broom plant.

somnus, i (fr. same root as Greek ὕπνος, sleep) sleep.

stim'ulus, i (cf. Greek στίζω, to prick up) prodding; stimulant.

stom'achus, i (fr. Gk. στόμα, mouth, and ἔχω, to receive) that which receives from the mouth, gullet, stomach.

succus, i (fr. *sugo*, to suck) juice.

sulcus, i (fr. same root as Greek ὀλκός, a trench) a ditch, groove.

syru'pus, i (Arabic *shcrab,* rose water) syrup.
cæcum, i (neuter of adj. *cæcus,* blind) blind gut.
cal'cium, i (fr. *calx,* lime) calcium.
cancrum, i (fr. *cancer,* a cancer) canker.
cap'sicum, i (fr. Greek *κάπτω,* to bite) Cayenne pepper.
centrum, i (fr. Greek *κέντρον,* a sharp point) a centre.
cera'tum, i (fr. *ccra,* wax) a cerate.
ce'rium, i (cf. *κηρίτης,* wax-stone) cerium.
cerebel'lum, i (dim. of *cerebrum*) the little brain.
cervix, i'cis (f) (allied to *κάρα,* head) neck.
ceta'ceum, i (*κῆτος,* a whale) spermaceti.
carbo, o'nis (m), charcoal, carbon.

EXERCISE XV.

A. 1. Medicus unciam tincturae catechu diarrhœae dat. 2. Sago et fructus rubi cibus sunt. 3. Chirurgus succum limonis arthritidi dat. 4. E succo sambuci (sumach) est color ruber. 5. Femina scirrhum mammae habet. 6. Scoparius et buchu sunt medicamenta (medicines) renibus et vesicae. 7. Fructus, limones et pyra medicamenta scorbuto sunt. 8. Syrupus papaveris somnum et soporem causat. 9. Alcohol est stimulus cerebri est systematis nervorum. 10. Vir octarium alcohol feminae dat.

B. 1. Bones have furrows, tuberosities and processes. 2. Syrup of hypophosphites is a medicine for wasting. 3. The blind gut and the stomach are in the belly. 4. The physician gives sulphide of calcium for carbuncles. 5. Oxalate of cerium is a remedy for vomiting. 6. Castor and valerian are stimulants of the nerves. 7. There is a gallon of alcohol in the shop. 8. Flowers of kousso and turpentine are remedies for tapeworm. 9. The man has a gallon of tincture of catechu, a pound of sago, and an ounce of sassafras. 10. The muscles and vessels of the neck.

CHAPTER XI.

DERIVATION OF NOUNS.

BY means of suffixes new nouns may be formed from the stems of other nouns, adjectives, or verbs.

I. Nouns derived from other nouns.

Diminutives. Diminutives denote a small thing of the kind specified by the original word; thus, from *cauda*, a tail, we have *caudicula*, a little tail. The gender of the derivatives thus formed is usually the same as that of the primitives. The following are the usual diminutive terminations:—

MASCULINE.	FEMININE.	NEUTER.
-ŭlus	-ŭla	-ŭlum
-cŭlus	-cŭlā	-cŭlum
-ŏlus	-ŏla	-ŏlum
-ellus	-ella	-ellum

Examples: *Lobus,* a lobe, *lobulus,* a little lobe, a lobule; *rana,* a frog, *ranula,* a little frog; *ovum,* an egg, *ovulum,* a little egg.

If the primitive is of the third, fourth, or fifth declensions, the diminutive is formed by adding *culus* or *iculus, a, um;* thus, *auris* (f), an ear, *auricula,* a little ear, external ear; *os* (n), a bone, *ossiculum,* a little bone (of ear); *funis* (m), a rope, *funiculus,* a little rope, a string, cord.

-olus and *-ellus, a, um,* are used in forming diminutives of all declensions; thus, *gladius,* a sword, *gladiolus,* a little sword; *modius,* a round measure, *modiolus,* a little cylindrical measure; *hordeum,* a barley corn, *hordeolum,* a little barley corn, a stye; *vita,* life, *vitellus,* a little life, yolk of an egg; *fons* (f), a fountain, *fontinella,* a little fountain (*fontenelle*).

Sometimes, when the diminutive makes a very long word it is contracted. The regular diminutive of *corona*, a crown, would be *coronella*, but that is shortened into *corolla*, a little crown, the colored part of a flower.

-arium added to the root of a noun denotes the place where the primitive abounds; thus, from *ovum*, an egg, we have *ovarium*, an egg basket, an ovary.

VOCABULARY XVI.

sac'culus, i (dim. of *saccus*, a bag) a little sack, saccule.

ventric'ulus, i (dim. of *venter*, the belly) a little belly,

infundib'ulum, i (dim. of *infundo*, a funnel) a little funnel.

mandib'ulum, i (dim. of *mando*, a glutton) little glutton; lower jaw-bone.

poc'ulum, i (dim. from πόω, to drink) a cup.

retinac'ulum, i (dim. form from *re*, back, *teneo*, to hold) retainer.

gubernac'ulum, i (dim. of *gubernator*, a pilot) a cord which guides the testis of the fœtus to the scrotum.

spec'ulum, i (dim. fr. *specio*, to look) a mirror, speculum.

spirac'ulum, i (dim. fr. *spiro*, to breathe) a small pore of the skin.

tenac'ulum, i (dim. fr. *teneo*, to hold) a small hook.

tuber'culum, i (dim. of *tuber*, a tuberosity) a tubercle.

vehic'ulum, i (dim. fr. *veho*, to carry) a vehicle.

vestib'ulum, i (dim. fr. *vestis*, a garment) the place where garments are taken off on entering a house; vestibule.

bicarbo'nas, a'tis (m) (from *bis*, twice, *carbo*, charcoal) bicarbonate.

bichro'mas, a'tis (m) (fr. *bis*, twice, *chromium*) bichromate.

bombax, a'cis (f) (from βόμβαξ, What the deuce is this?) cotton tree.

bubo, o'nis (m) (fr. Greek βουβων, the groin) an indurated inguinal gland.

buccina'tor, o'ris (m) (fr. *bucina,* a trumpet) a trumpeter; muscle of cheek.

cali'go, ig'inis (f) (kindred with *halo,* a mist) dimness of vision.

calx, calcis (m) (cf. Gk. χαλιξ, cement) lime.

canth'aris, idis (f) (Gk. κανθαρίς, a beetle) Spanish fly.

cor, cordis (n) (cf. Sansk. *hrid,* the heart) heart.

carbo'las, a'tis (m) (fr. *carbolicus,* carbolic) carbolate.

carbo'nas, atis (m) (fr. *carbo,* carbon) carbonate.

caro, carnis (f) (cognate with κρέας) flesh.

EXERCISE XVI.

A. 1. Cor auriculas et ventriculos habet. 2. Renes infundibula habent, mandibulum alveolos habet. 3. Syrupus aurantii vehiculum est. 4. In fœtu sunt gubernacula testum. 5. Tubercula in pulmonibus. 6. Chirrurgus specula et tenacula habet. 7. Medicus sodii benzoatem diphtheriae dat. 8. Borax cum melle est medicamentum cancro. 9. Bubones sunt aliquando symptomata syphilidis. 10. Musculi cordis non strias habet.

B. 1. The flesh of animals is food for men. 2. Bicarbonate of soda is a remedy for acid in the stomach. 3. Charcoal is a medicine for dyspepsia. 4. Gonorrhœa sometimes causes buboes. 5. The physician gives borax for aphthae. 6. The skin has hairs and perspiratory pores. 7. The lower jaw is a bone of the face. 8. The ear has a vestibule and small bones. 9. The boy has tubercles in his lungs. 10. A cup of water and a pint of alcohol.

II. *Nouns derived from adjectives.*

These are generally formed by adding *-etas, -itas, -tus,* or *-tudo,* all of the third declension, to the stem of the adjective. They are, as a rule, abstract nouns, and denote the condition of being expressed by the primitive like the English suffixes *ity, ty, tude,* and *ness.* Thus we may form from *levis,* light, *levitas,* lightness, levity; *acetus,* soured, *acetas,* sourness, acetate; *altus,* high, *altitudo,* height, altitude; *juvenis,* young, *juventus,* youth.

III. *Nouns derived from verbs.*

These are concrete nouns and are formed, usually, by adding *-or, -tor, -men* or *-mentum* to the stem of the verb.

-or, -oris, added to the stem of a supine, denotes that which performs the action expressed by the primitive; thus, from the supine *depressum,* from *deprimo,* to press down, we have *depressor,* that which presses down.

-men, -minis, denotes that to which the action expressed by the verb belongs; thus, from *fluo,* to flow, we have *flumen,* a flowing, a current.

-mentum, i, denotes the passive instrument of the action expressed by the verb; thus, from *ligo,* to bind, we get *ligamentum,* that by which a thing is bound, a ligament.

-tia æ is added to the stem of present participles and verbal adjectives to denote the quality expressed by the primitive, like English *ness, dom;* thus from *sapiens,* knowing, we have *sapientia,* knowledge.

-ura, added to the stem of a supine, denotes the thing resulting from the action expressed by the verb, or the thing which performs the action expressed by the verb. Thus, from *strictum,* supine of *stringo,* to contract, we have *strictura,* a stricture, the result of the contrac-

tion; from *fissum*, supine of *findo*, to split, is derived *fissura*, a fissure; and from *cinctum*, supine of *cingo*, to gird, we derive *cinctura*, a girdle, that which girds.

VOCABULARY XVII.

condimen′tum, i (fr. *condio*, to season) that with which a thing is seasoned.

corpus′culum, i (dim. of *corpus*, a body) corpuscle.

crassamen′tum, i (fr. *crasso*, to thicken) a clot.

elemen′tum, i (ety. unknown) an element.

fermen′tum, i (fr. *ferveo*, to ferment) a ferment.

frumen′tum, i (fr. *fruor*, to enjoy) grain; that by which we enjoy life.

herba′rium, i (fr. *herba*, a plant) a receptacle for plants.

ju′gulum, i (dim. of *jugum*, a yoke) little yoke, neck.

linimen′tum, i (fr. *lino*, to anoint) that with which we anoint.

omen′tum, i (from *ominor*, to foretell by omens) that by which we foretell, so called because the soothsayers examined the omentum and made their prophesies therefrom.

sanita′rium, i (from *sanitas*, health) a place where health abounds; a health resort.

pigmen′tum, i (from *pingo*, to paint) paint.

sarmen′tum, i (fr. *sarpo*, to creep) creepers of plants.

tegmen, inis (n) (fr. *tego*, to cover) a cover.

urna′rium, i (fr. *urna*, a funeral urn) a place where urns are kept.

vapo′rium, i (from *vapor*, steam) steaming department of Russian bath.

sanguis, inis (m) (allied to *sanus*, healthy) blood.

talus, i, the ankle bone, astragalus.

ter′minus, i (fr. τέρμα, a boundary) the end.

tarsus, i (Greek ταρσός, a basket) the ankle.

truncus, i (unknown) a trunk (of animal or tree).

trochis'cus, i (fr. Gk. τροχόω, to roll) a wheel, troche.

tu'bulus, i (dim. of *tubus*, a tube) a small tube.

ulmus, i (f) (ety. unknown) an elm tree.

umbili'cus, i (cf. ὀμφαλος, navel) navel.

u'terus, i (fr. *uter*, a bag made of skin) the womb.

ventus, i (perhaps from *venio*, to come, because always coming) wind.

virus,* i (n) (Sansk. *veshas* a filthy poison); virus.

EXERCISE XVII.

A. 1. Femina condimenta in cibo habet. 2. Corpuscula crassamenti et plasma sanguinis. 3. Aurum et cadmium elementa sunt. 4. Medicus spiritum frumenti viro dat. 5. Fermenta alcohol et acetum causant. 6. Linimentum cantharidis et aconiti. 7. Talus est os tarsi. 8. Anus est terminus intestini. 9. Trochisci ipecacuanhae et opii. 10. Levitas animi et sapientia aurum sunt.

B. 1. The tubules of the kidneys and of the testicles. 2. The poison of syphilis is in the blood. 3. The fœtus in the womb is in the fluid of the amnion. 4. The fibrin of the blood causes the clot. 5. He gives the man a drink of whisky. 6. There are ferments in the stomach. 7. A tumor of the ovary. 8. Troches of charcoal and bicarbonate of soda.

---

* *Virus* is the only neuter noun of the second declension, ending in *us*.

CHAPTER XII.

DECLENSION OF ADJECTIVES.

ADJECTIVES may be divided into two classes, according to their inflection: 1. Those belonging to the first and second declensions. 2. Those belonging to the third declension.

Adjectives agree with the nouns which they limit in gender, number, and case, consequently their terminations vary with the nouns to which they are attached.

I. *Adjectives of the first and second declensions.*

Adjectives of this class end in *us* or *er* in the nominative singular masculine, and are declined throughout in this gender like masculine nouns of the second declension; in the feminine they end in *a* and are declined like nouns of the first declension; in the neuter they end in *um* and are declined throughout like neuter nouns of the second declension.

Albus, white, is thus declined: —

SINGULAR.

	MASCULINE.	FEMININE.	NEUTER.
Nom.	albus	alba	album
Gen.	albi	albae	albi
Dat.	albo	albae	albo
Acc.	album	albam	album
Voc.	albe	alba	album
Abl.	albo	alba	albo

PLURAL.

	MASCULINE.	FEMININE.	NEUTER.
Nom.	albi	albae	alba
Gen.	albo'rum	alba'rum	albo'rum
Dat.	albis	albis	albis
Acc.	albos	albos	alba
Voc.	albi	albae	alba
Abl.	albis	albis	albis

In a similar manner are declined all adjectives ending in *us*, of this class.

VOCABULARY XVIII.

acer'bus, a, um (fr. *acer*, sharp) harsh, bitter.

acet'icus, a, um (fr. *acetum*, vinegar) acetic.

ac'idus, a, um (fr. *acco*, to be sour) acid.

acti'vus, a, um (fr. *ago*, to act) active.

Africa'nus, a, um (fr. Africa) African.

al'gidus, a, um (fr. *algeo*, to feel cold) chilly, cold.

ama'rus, a, um (fr. Sansk. *amas*, raw) bitter.

albus, a, um (cf. Greek ἀλφός, white leprosy) white.

anella'tus, a, um (fr. *anello*, to cover with rings) ringed.

anseri'nus, a, um (from *anser*, a goose) belonging to a goose.

anti'cus, a, um (fr. *ante*, before, place) anterior, front.

antiq'uus, a, um (fr. *ante*, before, time) ancient.

aquo'sus, a, um (fr. *aqua*, water) watery.

cartila'go, inis (f) (cf. from *caro*, flesh) cartilage, gristle.

chloras, a'tis (m) (tr. *chlorum*, chlorine) chlorate.

cica'trix, icis (f) (unknown) a scar.

bovi'nus, a, um (from *bos*, an ox) pertaining to cattle; bovine.

calcina'tus, a, um (fr. *calx*, lime) calcined; burnt to lime.

cal'idus, a, um (fr. *calor*, heat) warm.

A. 1. Uncia acidi acetici et drachma calcii sulphidi.   2. Cutis algida est cutis anserina.   3. Linea alba abdominis.   4. Status algidus cholerae Asiaticae.   5. Fructus quercus est amarus.   6. Trachea est tubus anellatus.   7. Musculi antici cervicis.   8. In artubus sunt ossa, cartilagines elasticae, et ligamenta.   9. Hippocrates medicus antiquus erat (was).   10. Cicatrix ab acie gladioli.

B. 1. A drachm of acetic acid.   2. The Spanish fly is an active medicine.   3. The surgeon cures the tumor and causes a scab.   4. Chloride of sodium is a salt.   5. The anterior muscle of the shin-bone.   6. The windpipe is ringed.   7. The body has flesh and white cartilages.   8. In vinegar there is acetic acid.   9. He gives bitter medicine for dyspepsia.

Adjectives of the first and second declensions ending in *er* in the nominative singular masculine are usually declined like *niger*, black (fr. root *nec*, to die, as seen in νεκρός, dead, *nox*, night, etc.: —

SINGULAR.

	MASCULINE.	FEMININE.	NEUTER.
Nom.	niger	nigra	nigrum
Gen.	nigri	nigrae	nigri
Dat.	nigro	nigrae	nigro
Acc.	nigrum	nigram	nigrum
Voc.	niger	nigra	nigrum
Abl.	nigro	nigra	nigro

PLURAL.

	MASCULINE.	FEMININE.	NEUTER.
Nom.	nigri	nigrae	nigra
Gen.	nigro'rum	nigra'rum	nigro'rum
Dat.	nigris	nigris	nigris
Acc.	nigros	nigras	nigra
Voc.	nigri	nigrae	nigra
Abl.	nigris	nigris	nigris

In a similar manner decline all adjectives of the first and second declensions ending in *er*, except *asper*, rough, *lacer*, torn, and *tener*, tender, which add the regular terminations to the nominative singular masculine; thus, *asper, aspera, asperum; asperi, asperæ, asperi*, etc.

VOCABULARY XIX.

æger, gra, grum (perhaps fr. *ἀ ἔργος*, not working) sick.

ater, tra, trum (fr. *ardeo*, to burn, *Dæderlein*) coal black.

creber, bra, brum (fr. *cresco*, to increase) frequent.

dexter, tra, trum (cf. Sanskrit *dekkan*, south, or *dhiu*, shining god) right hand.

glaber, bra, brum (cf. Greek *γλαφυρός*, smooth) without hair, smooth.

in'teger, gra, grum (*in*, not, *tango*, to touch or hurt) unhurt, whole.

macer, cra, crum (cf. *maceo*, to make soft or lean) lean, thin.

pulcher, chra, chrum (unknown) beautiful.

ruber, bra, brum (cf. *ἐρυθρός*, red) red.

sacer, cra, crum (fr. root *sac*; cf. Greek *ἅγ*, in, *ἅγιος*, holy) sacred, cursed.

scaber, bra, brum (cf. *scabo*, to scratch) rough, mangy.

sinis'ter, tra, trum (perhaps fr. *semi*, half, as in sinciput from *semi-caput*, because only half as skillful as the right) left hand.

calvus, a, um (cf. Germ. *kahl*, bald) bald.

can'didus, a, um (fr. *candco*, to be bright and white) shining white.

cani'nus, a, um (from *canis*, a dog) belonging to a dog; canine.

canus, a, um (kindred w. *xάω*, to burn) ash-colored, gray

caus'ticus, a, um (fr. Gk. *xάω*, to burn) burning, caustic.

cavus, a, um (kindred with *xάω*) burnt out hollow, empty.

nucha, æ (Arabic *nookah*, nape of neck) nape of neck.

chenopo'dium, i (Gk. *χήν*, a goose, *πούς*, a foot) goose foot

chlorofor'mum, i (fr. *chlorine* and *formyl*) chloroform.

cil'ium, i (kindred with *xύλις*, eyelid) eyelash.

col'chicum, i (from Greek *Xολχίτ*, Cholchis, where first obtained).

collo'dium, i (from *xόλλα*, glue) solution of gun-cotton in ether.

collum, i (cf. *cello*, to lift up) the neck.

coni'um, i (fr. Gk. *xωνείον*, hemlock) poison hemlock.

corian'drum, i (Greek *xορίαννον*, coriander) coriander.

creoso'tum, i (Gk. *xρέας*, meat, *σώζω*, to preserve) creosote

cuprum, i (fr. *Κύπρος*, Cyprus, where first obtained) copper

EXERCISE XIX.

A. 1. Virus bovinum vacciniam causat. 2. Superficies ossium cranii glabra est.   3. In viris ægris corpus macrum est.   4. Morbus sacer (epilepsy) os sacrum. 5. Os lineam asperam habet. 6. Rabies canina est morbus animalium.   7. In ære sunt acidum carbonicum, ammonia et vapor aquosus. 8. Liquor potassae causticus est. 9. Cranium est glabrum et cavum, facies rubra. 10. Chenopodium est medicamentum ascaridibus.

B. 1. The chloride of silver is white, sometimes black. 2. Chloroform causes anæsthesia. 3. The ligament of the nape of the neck. 4. Cayenne pepper is red;

the leaves are smooth. 5. Collodion is an etherial medicine. 6. The juice of hemlock. 7. In creosote there is carbolic acid. 8. The man has black eyelashes, hoary hair, and a red skin.

Some irregular adjectives of the first and second declensions. There are six adjectives ending in *us* and three in *er* in the nominative singular masculine, which form the genitive singular in *i'us* and the dative singular in *i* in all genders. In the plural they are regular.

Alius, other, is declined as follows:—

SINGULAR.

	MASCULINE.	FEMININE.	NEUTER.
Nom.	a'lius (Gk. ἀλλός)	a'lia	a'liud
Gen.	ali'us	ali'us	ali'us
Dat.	ali'i	ali'i	ali'i
Acc.	a'lium	a'liam	a'liud
Voc.	a'lie	a'lia	a'liud
Abl.	a'lio	a'lia	a'lio

The irregular adjectives given below are similarly declined, but have *um* regular in the neuter singular nominative and accusative.

VOCABULARY XX.

alter, era, erum (irreg.) (Greek ἀλλος, and, ἕτερος, other) the other.

neuter, tra, trum (irreg.) (non alter) neither.

nullus, a, um (irreg.) (*non ullus*, any) no; none.

ullus, a, um (irreg.) (fr. *unulus*, a little one) any.

unus, a, um (irreg.) (cf. Gk. ἕν, Ger. *ein*, Eng. *one*) one.

uter, tra, trum (irreg.) (perhaps fr. Gk. ὁπότερος) which of
    the two.

solus, a, um (irreg.) (perhaps fr. ὅλος, whole) sole, alone.

totus, a, um (irreg.) (unknown) whole.

aromat'icus, a, um (fr. Greek ἄρωμα, an odor) aromatic.

cine'reus, a, um (fr. *cinis,* ashes) ash-colored, ashy.

clarus, a, um (fr. same root as Ger. *klar*) clear, renowned.

clin'icus, a, um (fr. Greek κλίνη, a bed) clinical.

complex'us, a, um (from *cum,* together, and *plecto,* to
    weave) woven together; complex.

compos'itus, a, um (from *cum,* together, *pono,* to place)
    composite, compound.

conca'vus, a, um (from *cum,* completely, *cavus,* hollow)
    completely hollow; concave.

contu'sus, a, um (from *cum,* together, *tundo,* to break)
    bruised.

cauda'tus. a, um (fr. *cauda,* a tail) having a tail; caudate.

corrosi'vus, a, um (from *con,* intensive, *rodo,* to gnaw)
    corrosive.

crit'icus, a, um (fr. κρίνω, to decide) deciding; critical.

crucif'erus, a, um (fr. *crux,* a cross, *fero,* to bear) bearing
    a cross.

pars, partis (f) (fr. *pario,* to divide) a part, portion.

par, is (n) (unknown) equal; a pair.

hilum, i (cf. *nihilum,* nothing) a little thing; a seed point.

hydrar'gyrum, i (ὕδωρ, water, ἄργυρον, silver) quick-
    silver, mercury.

il'eum, i (fr. Gk. εἴλεος, twisted) third part small intestine.

il'ium, i (same as *ileum*) haunch bone.

EXERCISE XX.

A. 1. Medicus drachmam hydrargyri chloridi cor-
rosivi habet. 2. In officina est nullus acetas sodii.
3. Ileum pars intestini parvi. 4. Sunt duo (two) renes,

alter in dextra est, alter in sinistra. 5. Octarius tincturae gentianae compositae. 6. Spiritus ammoniae aro-
maticus est clavo medicamentum. 7. In abdomine est
axis cœliacus arteriarum. 8. Syrupus codeinae clarus
est. 9. In sanitate, color pulmonum cinereus est. 10. In
hepate sunt lobus caudatus et lobus Spigelii.

B. 1. The body is not the whole man. 2. Some
(*nonnullus*) things are of neither sex. 3. No man has
two lives. 4. One ounce of aromatic spirit of ammonia.
5. A gallon of carbonic acid. 6. The haunch-bone is a
part of the basin. 7. Bichlorides are corrosive salts.
8. The brain is a complex part of the body. 9. In the
head are pairs of nerves. 10. The whole body is the
work of nature.

II. Adjectives of the third declension.

Adjectives of the third declension may be divided
into three classes, according to the number of endings in
the nominative singular.

1. *Adjectives having three endings in the nominative
singular: er* masculine, *is* feminine, and *e* neuter.

Puter, rotten (from *puteo*, to stink) is declined as
follows:—

SINGULAR.

	MASCULINE.	FEMININE.	NEUTER.
Nom.	puter	putris	putre
Gen.	putris	putris	putris
Dat.	putri	putri	putri
Acc.	putrem	putrem	putre
Voc.	puter	putris	putra
Abl.	putri	putri	putri

PLURAL.

	MASCULINE	FEMININE.	NEUTER.
Nom.	putres	putres	pu'tria
Gen.	pu'trium	pu'trium	pu'trium
Dat.	pu'tribus	pu'tribus	pu'tribus
Acc.	putres	putres	pu'tria
Voc.	putres	putres	pu'tria
Abl.	pu'tribus	pu'tribus	pu'tribus

VOCABULARY XXI.

palus'ter, tris, tre (fr. *palus,* a swamp) marshy.

salu'ber, bris, bre (fr. *salus,* safety) safe, healthy.

sylves'ter, tris, tre (from *sylva,* a forest) growing with woods; sylvan.

vol'ucer, cris, cre (fr. *volo,* to fly) winged; flying.

curvus, a, um (fr. same root as κυρτός, crooked) curved.

despuma'tus, a, um (from *de,* out from, *spuma,* froth) clarified.

dilu'tus, a, um (fr. *dis,* apart, and *luo,* to wash) dilute.

diur'nus, a, um (fr. *dies,* a day) diurnal.

domes'ticus, a, um (fr. *domus,* a house) domestic.

dras'ticus, a, um (fr. Greek ὁράω, to be active) active.

durus, a, um (Sansk. *du,* to grieve, hurt) hard.

elas'ticus, a, um (from Greek ἐλαύνω, to drive) stretching, elastic.

elec'tricus, a, um (fr. ἤλεκτρον, amber, in which electricity was first observed) electric.

equi'nus, a, um (fr. *equus,* a horse) belonging to a horse; equine.

cydo'nium, i (from Κυδωνία, Cydonia, a city of Crete) a quince.

decoc'tum, i (fr. *de,* from, *coquo,* to cook) a decoction.

deliq'uium, i (from *deliquo*, to be lost) loss of conscious-
    ness; fainting.
delphin'ium, i (fr. Greek δελφίς, a dolphin) larkspur.
dorsum, i (cf. *retrorsum*, backward) the back.
dracon'tium, i (fr. δράκων, a dragon) skunk-cabbage.
efflu'vium, i (fr. *ex*, out, and *fluo*, to flow) a miasm.
elate'rium, i (fr. ἐλαύνω, to drive) elaterium.
emplas'trum, i (from ἐν, upon, and πλάσσω, to mould) a
    plaster.
extrac'tum, i (fr. *ex*, out, and *traho*, to draw) an extract.
cinis, ĕris (m) (cf. κάω, to burn, and κόνις, dust) ashes.
citras, ā'tis (m) (fr. *citrus*, a citron or lemon tree) citrate.
cortex, icis (m or f) (kindred with χορίον, leather) bark;
crus, cruris (n) (cf. κρέας, flesh) the leg.
dens, tis (m) (from same Aryan root as ὀδούς, a tooth) a
    tooth.
mors, mortis (m) (fr. *morior*, to die) death.

EXERCISE XXI.

A. 1. Decoctum corticis cinchonae rubrae. 2. Del-
phininum est planta palustris. 3. Fluxus sanguinis
deliquium animi causat. 4. Terra palustris non salubris
est. 5. Elaterium est medicamentum drasticum. 6. Acetum est acidum aceticum dilutum. 7. Viola et arum
sunt plantae sylvestres. 8. Cauda equina est terminus
medullae. 9. Emplastrum belladonnae, emplastrum cantharidis. 10. In mandibulo sunt dentes, in crure,
musculi.

B. 1. Syrup of bitter orange peel. 2. Death is
the end of the heart's labor. 3. The flexor muscles of
the leg. 4. The "hard mother" is a membrane of the
brain. 5. The cartilages of the vertebrae are elastic.
6. Dilute nitric acid and mustard plaster. 7. Clarified
honey is a vehicle for medicine. 8. The bloody matter

from rotting bone is putrid.   9. The ashes of the man's body are in the urnarium.   10. In swampy land there are effluvia and miasms.

---

2. *Adjectives of the third declension with two endings in the nominative singular.* Nearly all the adjectives of the third declension found in medical works are of of this variety, having *is,* for the termination of the nominative singular masculine and feminine, and *e* for the termination of the nominative singular neuter.

Dulcis, pleasant (from same root as Greek θέλγω, to please), is declined as follows:—

SINGULAR.

	MASC. AND FEM.	NEUTER.
Nom.	dulcis	dulce
Gen.	dulcis	dulcis
Dat.	dulci	dulci
Acc.	dulcem	dulce
Voc.	dulcis	dulce
Abl.	dulci or e	dulci or e

PLURAL.

	MASC. AND FEM.	NEUTER.
Nom.	dulces	dul'cia
Gen.	dul'cium	dul'cium
Dat.	dul'cibus	dul'cibus
Acc.	dulces	dul'cia
Voc.	dulces	dul'cia
Abl.	dul'cibus	dul'cibus

All adjectives of this variety are declined in a similar manner.

VOCABULARY XXII.

abdomina'lis, e (fr. *adomen*, the belly) abdominal.

abnor'mis, e (fr. *ab*, away from, and *norma*, a fixed rule) abnormal.

aborig'inis, e (fr. *ab*, from, *origo*, origin) original, aboriginal

acau'lis, e (fr. *a*, priv., and *caulis*, a stalk) stemless.

agres'tis, e (fr. *ager*, a field) growing in the fields.

ala'ris, e (fr. *ala*, a wing) winged, or wing-like.

alluvia'lis, e (from *ad*, against, *luo*, to wash) washed up, alluvial.

angula'ris, e (fr. *angulus*, an angle) angular.

annula'ris, e (fr. *annulus*, a little ring) ringed.

areola'ris, e (fr. *areola*, dim. of *area*, a vacant place) areolar

arsenica'lis, e (fr. *arsenicum*, arsenic) arsenical.

arteria'lis, e (fr. *arteria*, an artery) arterial.

arven'sis, e (from *arvum*, a cultivated field) growing in the fields.

austra'lis, e (fr. *auster*, the south wind) southern.

auricula'ris, e (fr. *auricula*, an auricle) auricular.

ebur, eb'oris (n), ivory.

erysip'elas, atis (m) (fr. Greek ἐρυθρός, red, πέλλας, skin) erysipelas.

falx, lcis (f) (Greek ϛαλκίϛ) a sickle, hook; process of dura mater.

femur, oris (n) (fr. *fero*, to bear) the thigh.

filix, icis (m) (fr. *felix*, fruitful, fertile) a fern.

flos, o'ris (m) (kindred with ϛλόος, blooming) a flower.

fomes, itis (m) (from *foveo*, to kindle) kindling material; contagium.

fons, ntis (m) (fr. *fundo*, to pour out) a fountain.

EXERCISE XXII.

A.   1. Octarius spiritus ætheris dulcis.   2. Aorta abdominalis est vas arterialis.   3. Plantae agrestes sunt

aliquando acaules. 4. Os cranii processus alares habet.
5. Terra alluvialis est locus filicibus. 6. Vertebrae processus arciformes et spinas habent. 7. Liquor arseni-
calis est medicamentum choreae. 8. Sanguis arterialis
est ruber. 9. Chirurgus tumores abnormes cuiat.
10 Appendices auriculares cordis.

B. 1. A portion of a tooth is ivory. 2. The sickle
of the brain is a process of the "hard mother." 3. The
flexor muscles of the thigh. 4. The edge of the angular
processes of the frontal bone. 5. Male fern causes the
death of tapeworms. 6. A gallon of tincture of arnica
flowers. 7. Arterial blood has no carbonic acid. 8. The
crowfoot growing in the fields is a beautiful flower.
9. In the tunic of the doctor is the contagious material
of cholera. 10. A drachm of sweet spirit of nitre.

---

3. *Adjectives of the third declension having but one
ending for all genders in the nominative singular.* The
adjectives of this class all end in *l*, *r*, *s*, or *x*, and increase
in the genitive. The present participle ending in *ns*
belongs to this class.

Ferox, fierce (from same root as *ferus*, wild) is declined as follows:—

SINGULAR.

	MASC. AND FEM.	NEUTER.
Nom.	ferox	ferox
Gen.	fero'cis	fero'cis
Dat.	fero'ci	fero'ci
Acc.	fero'cem	ferox
Voc.	ferox	ferox
Abl.	fero'ci or e	fero'ci or e

PLURAL.

	MASC. AND FEM.	NEUTER.
Nom.	fero'ces	fero'cia
Gen.	fero'cum	fero'cum
Dat.	feroc'ibus	feroc'ibus
Acc.	fero'ces	fero'cia
Voc.	fero'ces	fero'cia
Abl.	feroc'ibus	feroc'ibus

VOCABULARY XXIII.

attol'lens (fr. *ad*, up to, *tollo*, to raise) raising up.

at'rahens (fr. *ad*, to, and *traho*, to draw) drawing to.

ardens (fr. *ardeo*, to burn) burning; ambitious.

astrin'gens (fr. *ad*, to, *stringo*, to press) pressing together, astringent.

demul'cens (fr. *de*, from, *mulceo*, to strip) demulcent.

fervens (fr. *ferveo*, to boil) boiling.

fragrans (fr. *fragro*, to emit an odor) fragrant.

oppo'nens (from *ob*, against, *pono*, to place) opposing.

ret'rahens (fr. *re*, back, *traho*, to draw) retracting.

repens (fr. *repo*, to creep) creeping.

serpens (fr. *serpo*, to crawl like a snake) creeping.

semper'virens (fr. *semper*, ever, *virens*, green) evergreen.

tremens (fr. *tremo*, to tremble) trembling.

bilia'ris, e (fr. *bilis*, bile) biliary.

borea'lis, e (fr. Βόρεας, *Boreas*, the north wind) northern.

brachia'lis, e (fr. Greek βραχίων, the arm) brachial.

brevis, e (fr. same root as βραχύς, short) short.

bul'liens (fr. *bullio*, to boil) boiling.

campes'tris, e (fr. *campus*, a plain) growing in a plain.

canaden'sis, e (fr. *Canada*) Canadian.

capita'lis, e (fr. *caput*, the head) capital.

castren'sis, e (fr. *castra*, a camp) of inhabited places.

cauda'lis, e (fr. *cauda*, a tail) caudal.

cellula'ris, e (fr. *cellula,* dim. of *cella,* store-room) cellular.

centra'lis, e (fr. *centrum,* a centre) central.

cerea'lis, e (fr. *Ceres,* the goddess of the harvest) belonging to grain; cereal.

cervica'lis, e (fr. *cervix,* the neck) cervical.

columna'ris, e (fr. *columna,* a column, fr. *cello,* to raise) columnar.

commu'nis, e (from *con,* together, and *munus,* function) serving together, common.

cordia'lis, e (fr. *cor,* the heart) cordial, comforting.

ferrum, i (perhaps kindred with ἱερός (*hierus*), sacred. We see the opposite change in Spanish *hierro,* from *ferrum*) iron.

filtrum, i (from Old German *filt,* felt, of which filters were first made).

fluo'rium, i (fr. *fluor,* because assisting in the smelting of other metals) fluorine.

frænum, i (unknown) a check-rein, curb.

fulcrum, i (fr. *fulcio,* to prop) a prop.

gelse'mium, i (fr. Persian *yasamin,* jasmine) jasmine.

gera'nium, i (fr. Gk. γεράνιον, a little crane) cranesbill.

gossyp'ium, i (first found in Pliny) cotton root.

granum, i (Aryan *gar,* corn) a grain of corn; 1-60 of a drachm.

homo, minis (m) (fr. *humus,* the ground) mankind.

EXERCISE XXIII.

A. 1. In vesica biliare sunt calculi. 2. Musculus brachialis anticus est flexor cubiti. 3. Flexor brevis digitorum est musculus cubiti. 4. Granum extracti geranii. 5. Potus alcohol crebri sunt causa delirii trementis. 6. Typhus est morbus castrensis. 7. Os femoris est fulcrum cruris. 8. Fraenum linguae. 9. Gutta tincturae gelsemii sempervirentis. 10. In pulmonibus sunt tubuli bronchiales.

B. 1. The leaves of cranesbill are fragrant. 2. Fluorine is a chemical element. 3. There is boiling water
in the filter. 4. A salt of iron in the blood. 5. Tincture
of opium is a cordial. 6. The root of the cotton plant
causes abortion. 7. The raising muscle of the ear.
8. The scientific name of man is *homo sapiens.* 9. The
leaves of creeping triticum. 10. Cereal foods.

The present participle ending is *ns* forms the genitive in *ntis.*

Dolens, paining or painful, from *dolco,* to be in pain,
is declined as follows: —

SINGULAR.

	MASCULINE.	FEMININE.
Nom.	dolens	dolens
Gen.	dolen'tis	dolen'tis
Dat.	dolen'ti	dolen'ti
Acc.	dolen'tem	dolens
Voc.	dolens	dolens
Abl.	dolen'te or e	dolen'te or i

PLURAL.

	MASCULINE	FEMININE.
Nom.	dolen'tes	dolen'tia
Gen.	dolen'tium	dolen'tium
Dat.	dolen'tibus	dolen'tibus
Acc.	dolen'tes	dolen'tia
Voc.	dolen'tes	delen'tia
Abl.	dolen'tibus	dolen'tibus

11

CHAPTER XIII.

COMPARISON OF ADJECTIVES.

IN Latin, as in English, there are three degrees of comparison: the *positive*, the *comparative*, and the *superlative*.

The *comparative* degree is regularly formed by adding *ior* to the stem of the positive; thus, from *mitis*, mild, we have the comparative *mitior*, milder.

The *superlative* degree is regularly formed by adding *issimus, a, um* to the stem of the positive. Thus, from *mitis*, mild, we have the superlative *mitissimus*, mildest. When the nominative singular, however, ends in *er*, the superlative degree is formed by adding *rimus* to the positive; thus, from *ruber*, red, we have the superlative *ruberrimus, a, um*, reddest.

Adjectives of the comparative degree all belong to the third declension. For example, *fortior*, stronger, from *fortis*, strong, is thus declined: —

SINGULAR.

	MASC. AND FEM.	NEUTER.
Nom.	for'tior	for'tius
Gen.	fortio'ris	fortio'ris
Dat.	fortio'ri	fortio'ri
Acc.	fortio'rem	for'tius
Voc.	for'tior	for'tius
Abl.	fortio'ri or e	fortio'ri or e

PLURAL.

	MASC. AND FEM.	NEUTER.
Nom.	fortio'res	fortio'ra
Gen.	fortio'rum	fortio'rum
Dat.	fortior'ibus	fortior'ibus
Acc.	fortio'res	fortio'ra
Voc.	fortio'res	fortio'ra
Abl.	fortior'ibus	fortior'ibus

Adjectives of the superlative degree are declined like those of the first and second declensions.

VOCABULARY XXIV.

falsus, a, um (fr. past part. of *fallo,* to deceive) false.

febrif'ugus, a, um (from *febris,* fever, and *fugo,* to drive away) febrifuge.

feli'nus, a, um (fr. *felis,* a cat) feline.

flavus, a, um (cf. *φλόξ,* a flame) yellow.

flor'idus, a, um (fr. *flos,* a flower) blooming.

flu'idus, a, um (fr. *fluo,* to flow) fluid.

fulvus, a, um (allied to *flavus,* yellow) deep yellow, tawny.

fusus, a, um (fr. part. of *fundo,* to pour out) melted, fused.

gal'licus, a, um (fr. *Galli,* the Gauls, or *galla,* a gall-nut) French, gallic.

gas'tricus, a, um (fr. Greek *γαστήρ,* the stomach) gastric.

gem'inus, a, um (kindred with *γαμέω,* to marry) twin.

glaucus, a, um (Greek *γλαυκός,* bright) shining gray.

gratus, a, um (kindred w. *χάρις,* dear) pleasing, grateful.

grav'idus, a, um (fr. *gravis,* heavy) full, pregnant.

hepat'icus, a, um (fr. Greek *ῆπαρ,* the liver) hepatic.

huma'nus, a, um (fr. *homo,* a man) pertaining to man.

hyber'nus, a, um (fr. *hiems,* winter) wintry.

ili'acus, a, um (fr. *ilium,* the haunch-bone) iliac.

corona'lis, e (fr. *corona,* a crown) coronal.

cortica'lis, e (fr. *cortex,* bark) bark or outer layer.

costa'lis, e (fr. *costa,* a rib) costal.

crura'lis, e (fr. *crus,* a leg) belonging to a leg, crural.

fornix, icis (m) (allied to *furca,* a fork) arch, connection.

frigus, goris (n) (fr. same root as *ῥῖγος,* cold) cold.

frons, frondis (f) (fr. same root as *frux,* fruit) a stem.

frons, frontis (f) (cf. Greek *ὀφρύς,* eyebrow) forehead.

genus, ĕris (n) (kind. w. *γεννάω,* to produce) a race, genus.

glans, glandis (f) (kindred w. βάλανος, an acorn) a gland.

gluten, inis (n) (fr. *gluo*, to stick together) glue, gluten.

halo, ō'nis (f) (Gk. ἅλως, a circle around the sun) areola of nipple.

helix, ĭcis (f) (ἕλιξ, a coil) part of external ear.

herpes, ē'tis (m) (from ἕρπω, *serpo*, to creep) an eruptive skin disease.

hiru'do, ĭnis (f) (unknown) a leech.

hydrops, ō'pis (n) (from Greek ὕδωρ, water, ὤψ, looking) dropsy.

> **quam,** than.

EXERCISE XXIV.

A. 1. Diarrhœa est morbus mitior quam cholera. 2. Alcohol fortius est antisepticum. 3. Spinae vertebrarum ligamenta flava habent. 4. Extractum cornus floridae fluidum. 5. Potassa fusa est caustica. 6. Spiritus frumenti fortior est quam aqua. 7. Nervi craniales in paribus sunt. 8. Uterus abactus (empty) brevior est quam uterus gravidus. 9. In osse frontis sunt cavitates, in cerebro, fornix. 10. Gluten cereale est cibus diabeticorum.

B. 1. The surgeon has leeches and apparatus. 2. Dropsy of the amnion is not a common disease. 3. The "coil" of the ear and the gland of the penis. 4. The cat tribe, the dog species. 5. The bone of the forehead is a part of the skull. 6. There is the stem of a leaf in the fountain of water. 7. Cold is astringent, heat is antiseptic. 8. The "bark" of the brain and kidneys. 9. The iliac arteries and nerves. 10. Whisky is more pleasant than compound tincture of gentian.

IRREGULAR COMPARISON OF ADJECTIVES.

Many adjectives in Latin, as in the modern languages, are compared irregularly. This results from the use of synonyms, of which a part have been lost, so that the different degrees are often derived from entirely different words.

In the following list will be found the principal irregular adjectives used in medical works:—

POSITIVE.	COMPARATIVE.	SUPERLATIVE.
Bonus, *good*	me'lior,	op'timus
Dexter, *on the right*	dexte'rior	dex'timus
Ex'tera (f), *outward*	exte'rior	extre'mus
	infe'rior, *lower*	in'fimus
	inte'rior, *inner*	in'timus
Malus, *bad*	pejor	pes'simus
Magnus, *large*	major	max'imus
Multus, *many*	plus	plu'rimus
Parvus, *small*	minor	min'imus
Pos'tera, *behind*	poste'rior	postre'mus
	prior, *former*	primus
	pro'prior, *nearer*	prox'imus
Su'perus, *above*	supe'rior	supre'mus
	ulte'rior, *further*	ul'timus

When *quam*, than, is not expressed after the comparative degree, the noun with which the first thing is compared is put in the ablative case; thus we may say:— *Mel dulcius est quam acetum*, honey is sweeter than vinegar, or, *mel dulcius est aceto.*

The superlative is often rendered by the positive with *very;* thus *optimus vir* may be rendered either *the best man*, or *a very good man, an exceedingly good man.*

VOCABULARY XXV.

impu rus, a, um (fr. *im*, not, and *purus*, pure) impure.

in'dicus, a, um (fr. *India*) Indian.

innomina tus, a, um (fr. *in*, not, and *nomino*, to name) not named.

insa'nus, a, um (fr. *in*, not, and *sanus*, healthy) insane.

lac'ticus, a, um (fr. *lac*, milk) lactic.

largus, a, um, broad, large.

liq uidus, a, um (fr. *liquor*, a fluid) liquid.

longus, a, um (cf. Greek λογγάζω, to loiter) long.

latus, a, um (kindred with πλατύς, broad) broad, wide.

lotus, a, um (fr. *luo*, to wash) washed.

lymphat'icus, a, um (fr. *lympha*, clear water, lymph) lymphatic.

denta'tus, e (fr. *dens*, a tooth) toothed.

dorsa lis, e (fr. *dorsum*, the back) dorsal.

erec tilis, e (fr. *erigo*, to erect) erectile.

facia lis, e (fr. *facies*, the face) facial.

feb rilis, e (fr. *febris*, fever) febrile.

femora'lis, e (fr. *femur*, the thigh) femoral.

flex'ilis, e (fr. *flecto*, to bend) bending, flexile.

fœta'lis, e (fr. *fœtus*, an embryo) fœtal.

frag ilis, e (fr. *frango*, to break) easily broken, fragile.

nasus, i (cf. Aryan *sna*, to discharge, Eng. *snot*) the nose.

nastur tium, i (fr. *nasus*, nose, and *torqueo*, to twist) nasturtium.

infu sum, i (fr. *in*, in, and *fundo*, to pour) an infusion.

insec tum, i (fr. *in*, not, *seco*, to cut, too small to be cut) an insect.

intesti'num, i (fr. *intus*, within) intestine, gut.

io'dum, i (fr. ἰώδης, violet color) iodine.

ka'lium, i (fr. Arabic *kali*, an alkaline plant) potassium.

la'bium, i (perhaps fr. *labor*, to slip or slide) lip.

labrum, i (fr. *labium*, a lip) the lip of a flower or insect.

lactuca'rium, i (fr. *lac*, milk, the color of its juice) lettuce.

lardum, i (cf. Greek λαρός, fat) lard.

lignum, i (kindred with *ligo*, to bind) fire wood, wood.

linum, i (Greek λίνον, flax) flax.

lith'ium, i (fr. Greek λίθος, a stone) lithium.

A. 1. Musculi faciales et dorsales multi sunt. 2. Musculus longissimus dorsi major est longo muculo colli. 3. Libra sulphuris loti et drachma nasturtii gemmarum. 4. In vulva feminae sunt labia majora et minora. 5. Tinctura cannabis Indicae est stimulus nervorum. 6. Levatores labii superioris sunt musculi ' faciales. 7. Musculus latissimus dorsi est depressor acromii. 8. Infusum lactucarii soporem causat. 9. In vagina sunt labia et cervix uteri. 10. Caput foetale maris majus est quam caput foetale femininum.

B. 1. Quinine and aconite are very good medicines for febrile diseases. 2. River water is good for drinking and baths. 3. The bones of birds are more fragile than those of cats and dogs. 4. The outer surface of the frontal bone is smooth. 5. The small gut is longer than the large. 6. Infusion of digitalis is a medicine for diseases of the heart. 7. The extending muscle of the "smallest" (little) finger. 8. The physician gives a flax seed poultice to the boy. 9. Carbonate of lithium is diuretic. 10. Itch is a bad disease, syphilis is worse, but leprosy the worst of all.

CHAPTER XIV.

NUMERAL ADJECTIVES.

NUMERAL * adjectives are of three kinds, viz., cardinals, ordinals, and distributives. From numeral adjectives numeral adverbs are derived.

CARDINALS.	ORDINALS.	DISTRIBUTIVES.	NUMERAL ADVERBS.
Unus, j	primus, *first*	sin'guli, *one by one*	semel, *once*
Duo, ij	secun'dus, *second*	bini, *two by two*	bis, *twice*
Tres, iij	ter'tius, *third*, etc.	terni, *three by three*	ter, *thrice*
Quatuor, iv	quartus	quater'ni	quater, *four times*
Quinque. v	quintus	quini	quin'quies
Sex, vj	sextus	seni	sex'ties
Septem, vij	sep'timus	septe'ni	sep'ties
Octo, viij	octa'vus	octo'ni	oc'ties
Novem, ix	nonus	nove'ni	no'nies
Decem, x	dec'imus	deni	de'cies
Un'decim, xj	undec'imus	unde'ni	unde'cies
Duod'ecim, xij	duodec'imus	duode'ni	duode'cies
Tre'decim, xiij	ter'tius dec'imus	terni deni	terde'cies
Quatuor'decim, xiv	quartus dec'imus	quater'ni deni	quatuorde'cies
Quin'decim, xv	quintus dec'imus	quini deni	quinde'cies
Se'decim, xvj	sextus dec'imus	seni deni	sede'cies
Septen'decim. xvij	sep'timus dec'imus	septe'ni deni	de'cies et sep'ties
Vigin'ti, xx	vices'simus	vice'ni	vi'cies
Quinquagin'ta, l	quinquages'simus	quinquage'ni	quinqua'gies
Centum, c	centes'simus	cente'ni	cen'ties
Mille, m	milles'simus	mille'ni	mil'lies

---

* *Numerus*, a number, comes from an Aryan root, *nam*, meaning to divide. It may interest the student to know that the names of numerals in all languages are derived by metaphor. Thus, *one*, Greek *hen*, Latin *unus*, and German *ein*, are all derived from the root of the first personal pronoun *I*. The word *two*, Greek and Latin *duo*, is from the root of the second personal pronoun, cf. German *Du*, Greek and Latin *te*, *tuus*. *Five*, Greek *pente*, Latin *quinque*, German *fuenf*, are all akin to the Sansk. *pani*, the hand, which has five fingers. The Greek *deca*, ten, and Latin *decem*, contain the same root as the Greek *dactylos* and Latin. *digitus*, finger, the ten fingers being thus the foundation of the decimal system.

Unus, one, is declined throughout, of course only in the singular, like an irregular adjective of the first and second declensions. (See declension of *alius*, p. 141.)

Duo, two, is declined as follows:—

	MASCULINE.	FEMININE.	NEUTER.
Nom.	duo	duae	duo
Gen.	duo'rum	dua'rum	duo'rum
Dat.	duo'bus	dua'bus	duo'bus
Acc.	duos or o	duas	duo
Voc.	duo	duae	duo
Abl.	duo'bus	dua'bus	duo'bus

Tres, three, is declined like an adjective of two endings of the third declension; thus, *tres, tria; trium, trium*, etc. All other cardinals are indeclinable.

Ordinals are declined like adjectives of the first and second declensions.

Distributives are declined like adjectives of the first and second declensions in the plural, but form the genitive masculine and neuter in *um* instead of *o'rum;* thus, masculine *bini*, feminine *binae*, neuter, *bina*, nominative; *binum, binarum, binum*, genitive, etc.

There is also a class of *multiplicatives* ending in *plex* from *plico*, to fold; thus, *simplex (semelplex)* single, *duplex*, double, *triplex*, triple, *quadruplex*, fourfold, etc.

VOCABULARY XXVI.

or'ganum, i (fr. Greek ὀργέω, to work) a tool, organ.
os'tium, i (fr. *os*, a mouth) an entrance.
ox'idum, i (fr. ὀξύς, sour) an oxide.
pab'ulum, i (fr. *pascor*, to graze) fodder, nutriment.
pala'tum, i (fr. *balato*, to bleat) the palate.
palla'dium, i (fr. Παλλάς, Minerva) the metal palladium.

pedilu'vium, i (fr. *pedes*, feet, and *luo*, to wash) foot bath.

plumbum, i (cognate with μόλυβδος lead) lead.

podophyl'lum, i (fr. Greek πούς, foot, and φύλλον, leaf) mandrake.

potas'sium, i (fr. English *potash*) also called *kalium*.

poma'tum, i (fr. *pomum*, fruit) a pommade.

index, icis (m) (fr. *indico*, to point out) first finger.

iter, in'eris (n) (fr. *ire*, to go) a passage.

jecur, ŏris (m) (cognate with ἧπαρ) liver.

jus, juris (n) (cf. *jugum*, a yoke) that which is binding, law.

lac, lactis (m) (cognate with γάλα, milk) milk.

lanu'go, ĭnis (f) (fr. *lana*, wool) downy hair on skin.

lens, tis (f) (unknown) a lentil, lens.

lien, ĕnis (n) (cognate with σπλήν, spleen) spleen.

lues, luis (f) (cf. λυγρός, baneful) pestilence, syphilis.

lumba'go, inis (f) (fr. *lumbus*, the loin) lumbago.

opa'cus, a, um (fr. ὀπός, juice) juice colored, opaque.

op'ticus, a, um (fr. ὄπτω, to see) optic.

oxal'icus, a, um (fr. ὀξαλίς, sorrel) oxalic.

pal'lidus, a, um (fr, *palleo*, to be pale) pallid.

pathet'icus, a, um (fr. πάθος, feeling, emotion, disease) pathetic.

paucus, a, um (kindred with *parum*, little) few.

planus, a, um (fr. contract. of *placnus*, Germ. *platz*, an open place) level.

posti'cus, a, um (fr. *postea*, behind) posterior.

purus, a, um (fr. a root *pu*, meaning to clean) pure.

muli'ebris, e (fr. *mulier*, a woman) belonging to woman.

nob'ilis, e (fr. *gnosco*, to know) learned, noble.

occidenta'lis, s (fr. *occidens*, settling down of the sun) western.

EXERCISE XXVI.

A. 1. Homo, jecinorem unum, lentes duas, et organa multa habet. 2. Patheticus est nervus quartus cranii.   3. Pilulae duae ter in die.   4. Lumbago est neuralgia musculorum dorsalium.   5. Nervus opticus est nervus secundus cranii.   6. In cranio sunt ossa octo, in facie quatuordecim.   7. Nervi tertii, quarti et sexti cranii sunt motores oculi.   8. Portio mollis nervi septimi cranialis est nervus auditorius.   9. Peroneus tertius est musculus cruris.   10. Plumbum est metallum grave.

B.   1. Oleoresin of mandrake.   2. In the forearm is the long flexor of the first finger.   3. The eight bones of the carpus.   4. The third bone of the little finger. 5. The plane bone of the orbit.   6. Oxalic acid is bitter. 7. In sour milk there is lactic acid.   8. There are two hundred bones in the body.

CHAPTER XV.

DERIVATION OF ADJECTIVES.

DERIVATIVE adjectives are formed principally from nouns and verbs.

1. *Adjectives derived from nouns are called denomitives,* and are formed by adding suffixes to the stem of the noun.

-eus, a, um, and *-inus, a, um,* denote material or resemblance, like the English suffixes *ous* and *en.*

Examples: *Aureus,* golden, from *aurum,* gold; *piceus,* pitchy, from *pix,* pitch; *adaman'tinus,* adamantine, from *adamas,* adamant.

-a'lis, e; -a'ris, e; -a'rius, a, um; -o'rius, a, um; -i'lis, e; -at'ilis, e; -ic'ius, a, um; -icus, a, um; -ius, a, um; -i'nus, a, um. The above suffixes signify belonging or pertaining to the thing denoted by the noun.

Examples: *Fœtalis,* pertaining to the fœtus; *alaris,* pertaining to a wing; *salivarius,* pertaining to spittle; *tinctorius,* pertaining to dyers; *senilis,* pertaining to an old man; *saxatilis,* belonging to the rocks; *patricius,* belonging to the father; *pulmonicus,* belonging to a lung; *vesicatorius,* pertaining to a blister; *equinus,* pertaining to a horse.

Observation: The termination *-inus, a, um* belongs especially to animals. Thus, we have *felinus,* feline, cat-like; *elephantinus,* from *elephas.*

-o'sus, a, um; -len'tus, a, um, denote abounding in the thing expressed by the noun.

Examples: *Nervosus,* abounding in nerves; *virulentus,* abounding in poison.

-en'sis, e; -a'nus, a, um, attached to the stems of the names of places, denote belonging to a place.

Examples: *Chinensis,* belonging to China; *Virginianus,* belonging to Virginia.

-a'tus, a, um, denotes furnished with the thing designated by the noun.

Examples: *Barbatus,* having a beard; *pinnatus,* having wings; *vertebratus,* furnished with vertebræ; *venenatus,* furnished with poison; *cornutus,* furnished with horns.

2. *Adjectives derived from verbs are called verbals,* and are usually formed by means of the following suffixes:—

-bundus, a, um, added to the stem of a verb, has a strengthened meaning of the present participle in *us,* English *ing.*

Example: From *morior,* to die, we have *moribundus,* about to die, moribund.

-idus, a, um; -uus, a, um, added to the stems of neuter verbs to denote the quality expressed by the verb.

Examples: From *valeo,* to be of worth, *validus,* of value; from *noceo,* to be harmful, *noccuus,* injurious.

-ilis, e; -bilis, e, added to the stem of a verb, denote capability or desert.

Examples: From *duco,* to lead or draw, *ductilis,* capable of being drawn; from *retraho,* to retreat, *retractilis,* capable of being drawn back; from *texo,* to weave, *textilis,* capable of being woven; from *volo,* to fly away, *volatilis,* capable of flying away; from *horreo,* to frighten, *horribilis,* capable of frightening.

-a'tus, -e'tus, -itus, i'tus, terminations of past participles, equivalent to English *-ed.*

Examples: *Perfero,* to perforate. *perforatus,* perforated; *acco,* to be sour, *acetum,* soured; *sulco,* to be accustomed, *solitus*, accustomed; *partio*, to divide, *partitus*, divided.

-*ns* is the termination of present participle, English -*ing;* thus, from *repo*, to creep, *repens*, creeping.

VOCABULARY XXVII.

cosmet'icus, a, um (fr. Greek κοσμέω, to adorn) cosmetic.

grac'ilis, e (Sanskrit *gca*, thin) slender, graceful.

gravis, e (cognate with βαρύς, heavy) heavy.

iner'mis, e (*in*, without, *arma*, arms) unarmed.

inguina'lis, e (fr. *inguen*, the groin) inguinal.

intercosta'lis, e (from *inter*, between, *costa*, rib) between the ribs.

interspina'lis, e (fr. *inter*, between, *spina*, spine) between the spinous processes.

jugula'ris, e (fr. *jugulum*, the neck) jugular.

lactea'lis, e (fr. *lac*, milk) lacteal.

letha'lis, e (fr. Gk. λήθη, the river from which the souls of the dead drank causing them to forget the past) deadly.

mala'ris, e (fr. *mala*, the cheek) malar.

margina'lis, e (fr. *margo*, a border) marginal.

mola'ris, e (fr. *mola*, a millstone) molar (tooth).

morta'lis, e (fr. *mors*, death) deadly.

matu'rus, a, um (kindred with *mater*, mother) ripe.

media'nus, a, um (fr. *medius*, middle) median.

mor'bidus, a, um (fr. *morbus*, a disease) diseased.

novus, a, um (cognate with νέος, new) new.

obliq'uus, a, um (from *ob*, against, and a root *lak*, to lean) slanting.

lycopo'dium, i (fr. λύκος, a wolf, πούς, foot) wolf's foot.

meco'nium, i (fr. μήκων) poppy juice) contents of fœtal intestine.

membrum, i (kind. w. *membrana,* a membrane) member.
men'struum, i (fr. *mensis,* monthly purgation) a vehicle
  or solvent.
mollus'cum, i (fr. *mollis,* soft) a mollusc.
momen'tum, i (fr. *moveo,* to move) moving force.
monstrum, i (fr. *moneo,* to warn) evil omen; a monstrosity
o'leum, i (fr. *oliva,* olive, fr. which *oleum* was obtained) oil.
crista, æ (fr. same root as *crinis,* hair) crest, topknot.
gallus, i (fr. root *gar,* to call *garlus*) a cock.

EXERCISE XXVII.

A. 1. Epilepsia gravior est morbus horribilis.
2. Crista galli est pars ossis ethmoidalis. 3. Ossa crani-
alia immobilia sunt. 4. Tæniae sunt inermes, nanae,
latae, et sagittatae. 5. Bubo est inflammatio glandis
inguinalis. 6. Dosis lethalis opii est de granis tribus ad
grana viginti. 7. Os malare, dentes molares. 8. Vir est
homo masculus. 9. Columna spinalis est linea corporis
mediana. 10. Virus morbidum rabiem caninum causat.

B. 1. In the ovaries there are ovules, in the uterus
an egg. 2. In morbid poison there are pathogenetic
bacteria. 3. The external oblique muscle of the abdomen. 4. In the gut of the foetus there is meconium.
3. The virile member of a man. 6. Gold and silver have
I none. 7. Contagious mollusc is a disease of the skin.
8. Oil of clove and bitter almond. 9. The birth of a
monstrosity is a cause of tears. 10. Oleo-resin of male
fern.

CHAPTER XVI.

Pronouns.

THE regular third personal pronoun, *is, ea, id*, he, she, it, is seldom used in medical Latin, *idem, eadem, idem*, the same, being preferred.

Idem is declined as follows:—

SINGULAR.

	MASCULINE.	FEMININE.	NEUTER.
Nom.	idem	e'aden	idem
Gen.	ejus'dem	ejus'dem	ejus'dem
Dat.	ei'dem	ei'dem	ei'dem
Acc.	eun'dem	ean'dem	idem
Abl.	eo'dem	ea'dem	eo'dem

PLURAL.

	MASCULINE.	FEMININE.	NEUTER.
Nom.	ii'dem	eae'dem	e'adem
Gen.	eorun'dem	earun'dem	eorun'dem
Dat.	eis'dem	eis'dem	eis'dem
Acc.	eos'dem	eas'dem	e'adem
Abl.	eis'dem	eis'dem	eis'dem

The relative *qui, quae, quod*, who, which, is thus declined:—

SINGULAR.

	MASCULINE.	FEMININE.	NEUTER.
Nom.	qui	quae	quod
Gen.	cujus	cujus	cujus
Dat.	cui	cui	cui
Acc.	quem	quam	quod
Abl.	quo	qua	quo

PLURAL.

	MASCULINE.	FEMININE.	NEUTER.
Nom.	qui	quae	quae
Gen.	quorum	quarum	quorum
Dat.	quibus	quibus	quibus
Acc.	quos	quas	quae
Abl.	quibus	quibus	quibus

The demonstratives *hic, haec, hoc,* this (near us), and *ille, illa, illud,* that (yonder), like adjectives, agree with the nouns which they limit in gender number and case. When two things are mentioned *hic* is applied to the latter, and *ille* to the former; thus, *vir et puella, haec est pulchra, ille, fortis.* "The man and the girl, the latter is beautiful, the former brave."

SINGULAR.

	MASCULINE.	FEMININE.	NEUTER.
Nom.	hic	haec	hoc
Gen.	hujus	hujus	hujus
Dat.	huic	huic	huic
Acc.	hunc	hanc	hoc
Voc.	hic	haec	hoc
Abl.	hoc	hac	hoc

PLURAL.

	MASCULINE.	FEMININE.	NEUTER.
Nom.	hi	hae	haec
Gen.	horum	harum	horum
Dat.	his	his	his
Acc.	hos	has	haec
Voc.	hi	hae	haec
Abl.	his	his	his

SINGULAR.

	MASCULINE.	FEMININE.	NEUTER.
Nom.	ille	illa	illud
Gen.	illi'us	illi'us	illi'us
Dat.	illi	illi	illi
Acc.	illum	illam	illud
Voc.	ille	illa	illud
Abl.	illo	illa	illo

12

PLURAL.

	MASCULINE.	FEMININE.	NEUTER.
Nom.	illi	illae	illa
Gen.	illo'rum	illa'rum	illo'rum
Dat.	illis	illis	illis
Acc.	illos	illas	illa
Voc.	illi	illae	illa
Abl.	illis	illis	illis

VOCABULARY XXVIII.

cochlea're, is (n) (fr. Greek *κοχλίας*, a small shell) a shell, a spoon.

princip'ium, i (fr. *primum*, first *capio*, to take) a beginning.

puden'dum, i (future part. of *pudeo*, to be ashamed) of which one should be ashamed, genitalia.

punctum, i (fr. *pungo*, to prick) a point.

pyr'ethrum, i (fr. *πῦρ*, fire, fever, *ἐρυθρός*, red) "fever few."

quadriho'rium, i (from *quartus*, a fourth, *hora*, hour) a quarter of an hour.

rectum, i (fr. *rego*, to lead straight) straight, straightgut.

regnum, i (fr. *rego*, to lead) a reign, kingdom.

reme'dium, i (fr. *re*, again, *medeor*, to heal) a remedy.

rheum, i (fr. *Rha*, a name for the river Volga) rhubarb.

rostrum, i (fr. *rodo*, to gnaw or pick) a beak, muzzle.

scammo'nium, i (fr. Greek *σκαμμωνία*, bind-weed, from *σκάμβος*, crooked) scammony.

scrotum, i (cogn. w. *χόριον*, a hide) pouch, bag of a male.

matrix, i'cis (f) (fr. *mater*, mother) the nourishing part, womb, root.

mucila'go, inis (f) (fr. *mucus*, Gk. *μύχος*, mucus) mucilage.

nox, noctis (f) (from Aryan *nak*, destroy; cf. Greek *νύξ*, night) night.

nux, nucis (f) (kind. w. *nutrio*, to nourish) a nut, kernel.

præpara′tus, a, um (part. fr. *præparo,* prepare) prepared.
profun′dus, a, um (*pro,* out from, *fundus,* depth) deep.
purifica′tus (fr. *purus,* pure, *facio,* to make) made pure.
quadra′tus, a, um (fr. *quatuor,* four) square.
quantus, a, um (fr. *quam,* as) as much as.
quarta′nus, a, um (fr. *quartus,* fourth) belonging to the
fourth day.
quotidia′nus, a, um (fr. *quotidies,* every day) quotidian.
oc′ciput, itis (n) (fr. *ob,* opposite, *caput,* the head) base of
the head.
os, oris (f) (fr. Aryan *as,* to live, breathe) the mouth.
orbicula′ris, e (fr. *orbis,* a circle) circular.
orbita′lis, e (fr. *orbita,* the orbit, fr. *orbis,* a circle) orbital.
ova′lis, e (fr. *ovum,* an egg) egg-shaped.
palma′ris, e (fr. *palma,* the palm) palmar.
parieta′lis, e (fr. *paries,* a wall, fr. *pario,* to divide) parietal.
pectora′lis, e (fr. *pectus,* the chest, breast) pectoral.
peren′nis, e (fr. *per,* through, *annus,* the year) perennial,
living throughout the years.
planta′ris, e (fr. *planta,* the sole) plantar.
rec′ipe (verb) ((*re,* again, *capio,* to take) take (imperative)

EXERCISE XXVIII.

A. 1. Recipe cochleare medium cretae preparatae
nocte. 2. Pudenda maris sunt penis, pubes et scrotum.
3. In conjunctiva sunt puncta lachrymalia. 4. Recipe
cochleare magnum spiritus frumenti omni quadrihorio.
5. Rectum est pars tertia magni intestini. 6. Saccharum
lactis dulce est. 7. In naso est rostrum vomeris.
8. Oleum santali est remedium gonorrhœae. 9. Mucilago est vehiculum utile. 10. Flexor profundus digitorum est musculus cubiti.

B.   1. The square lobe of the liver.   2. The sick man has a daily fever.   3. The occipital bone is the lowest in the skull.   4. Compound pills of iron are officinal.   5. The circular muscles of the mouth.   6. In the orbit there are sutures, grooves, and fissures.   7. The oval hole of the fœtal heart.   8. The long palmar muscle is a flexor.   9. The plantar muscle is a flexor of the toes.   10. The violet and the rose are perennial plants.

CHAPTER XVII.

THE VERB.

A FULL discussion of the Latin verb is a subject outside of the province of this book. We will, accordingly, limit our study to those parts of the verb employed in prescription writing.

In the active voice, the imperative second person singular, and the subjunctive third person singular, are the only parts used.

In the passive voice, the infinitive, the third person singular subjunctive, the gerund or future participle, and past participle, are the only parts employed. For example, take *agita're*, to shake; we may use in the active voice the imperative *agita*, shake (thou), and the subjunctive third person singular, *agitet*, let him shake. In the passive voice we may use the infinitive *agitari*, to be shaken; the subjunctive third person singular, *agitetur*, let it be shaken; the gerund, *agitandus, -a, -um, (est)*, it should be shaken; and the past participle, *agitatus, -a, -um*, shaken.

1. *The Conjugations:* There are four conjugations or methods of inflecting the verb, depending upon the vowel which precedes the ending *re* of the present infinitive active.

Verbs whose present infinitive active ends in:—

> āre, are of the first conjugation.
> ēre, are of the second conjugation.
> ĕre, are of the third conjugation.
> īre, are of the fourth conjugation.

2. *The imperative active second person singular* is used in giving directions to the dispenser, and is formed by dropping the termination *re* of the infinitive.

> Examples: Agita′*re*, to shake (1st conj.) *ag′ita*, shake (thou).
> Admovē′*re*, to apply (2d conj.) *admo′ve*, apply (thou).
> Ad′dĕ*re*, to add (3d conj.) *ad′de*, add (thou).
> Parti′*re*, to divide (4th conj.) *parti*, divide (thou).

3. *The subjunctive active third person singular* is formed by adding the following terminations to the stem of the verb:—

> In the first conjugation, (et), thus, ag′itet, let him shake.
> In the second conjugation, (eat), thus, admove′at, let him apply.
> In the third conjugation, (at), thus, addat, let him add.
> In the fourth conjugation, (iat), thus, partiat, let him divide.

4. *The infinitive passive* is formed in all conjugations except the third by changing the final *e* of the infinitive active to *i.* Thus, *agitari*, to be shaken; *moveri*, to be moved, etc. In the third conjugation the infinitive passive is formed by adding *i* to the root, as *addi*, to be added.

5. *The passive of the subjunctive third person singular* is formed by adding *ur* to the subjunctive; thus, *agitet′ur*, let it be shaken, *admovea′tur*, let it be applied.

6. *The future passive participle or gerund* is formed in the four conjugations by adding to the stem of the verb, -*andus, -a, -um, -endus, -endus*, and -*iendus*, respectively; thus, *agitandus*, about to be shaken, *admovendus*, etc.

The uses of the different parts of the verb are illustrated in the following prescription:—

> Recipe,   Pulveris Jalapae compositae unciam,
>   Potassii Bitartratis uncias duas.
> Misce.   Ejusdem capiat æger cochleare parvum nocte maneque
>   donec anasarca curari videatur, dein præ-
>   scribe pilulas ferri compositas quarum duae
>   ter in die sumendae sunt.

VERBS OF THE FIRST CONJUGATION.

	ACTIVE VOICE.			PASSIVE VOICE.	
Infinit.	*Imp. 2d person sing.*	*Subj. 3d person sing.*	*Infinit.*	*Subjunct.*	*Gerund.*
Dare, *to give*	da, *give (thou)*	det, *let him give*	dari, *to be given*	detur, *let it be given*	dandus, *about to be given*
Colare, *to strain*	cola	colet	colari	coletur	colandus
Continuare, *to continue*	continua	continuet	cotinuari	continuetur	continuandus
Applicare, *to apply*	applica	applicet	applicari	applicetur	applicandus
Evaporare, *to evaporate*	evapora	evaporet	evaporari	evaporetur	evaporandus
Inhalare, *to inhale*	inhala	inhalet	inhalari	inhaletur	inhalandus
Macerare, *to macerate*	macera	maceret	macerari	maceretur	macerandus
Parare, *to prepare*	para	paret	parari	paretur	parandus
Potare, *to drink*	pota	potet	potari	poietur	potandus
Pulverare, *to powder*	pulvera	pulveret	pulverari	pulveretur	pulverandus
Purgare, *to purge*	purga	purget	purgari	purgetur	purgandus
Renovare, *to renew*	renova	renovet	renovari	renovetur	renovandus
Servare, *to keep*	serva	servet	servari	servetur	servandus
Signare, *to mark*	signa	signet	signari	signetur	signandus
Stare, *to stand*	sta	stet			
Usurpare, *to take*	usurpa	usurpet	usurpari	usurpetur	usurpandus

VERBS OF THE SECOND CONJUGATION.

	ACTIVE VOICE.			PASSIVE VOICE.	
Infinit.	*Imperat.*	*Subjunct.*	*Infinit.*	*Subjunct.*	*Gerund.*
Augere, *to increase*	auge, *increase*	augeat, *let him in-* [*crease*	augeri, *to be increased*	augeatur, *let it be in-* [*creased*	augendus, *about to be*
Cavere, *to avoid*	cave	caveat	caveri	caveatur	cavendus [*increased*
Ciere, *to excite*	cie	cieat	cieri	cieatur	ciendus
Exhibere, *to give*	exhibe	exhibeat	exhiberi	exhibeatur	exhibendus
Fovere, *to foment*	fove	foveat	foveri	foveatur	fovendus
Miscere, *to mix*	misce	misceat	misceri	misceatur	miscendus
Movere, *to stir*	move	moveat	moveri	moveatur	movendus
Respondeo, *to answer*	responde	respondeat	responderi	respondeatur	respondendus

VOCABULARY XXIX.

sebum, i (Sansk. *stavara*, hard fat) oily secretions of skin.

semicu'pium, i (*semi*, half, *cubo*, to lie down) a half bath, hip bath.

septum, i (fr. *sepio*, to fence in) a fence, partition.

seques'trum, i (fr. *sequor*, to follow) a remnant, piece of dead bone.

serum, i (cf. ὀρός, serum) watery part of milk or blood.

signum, i (fr. *signo*, to mark) a label, sign.

spectrum, i (fr. *specio*, to look) an image.

sputum, i (fr. *spuo*, to spit) spittle.

stannum, i (*stagnum*, an alloy of silver and lead) tin.

sternum, i (Greek στέρνον, breast-bone) breast-bone.

stib'ium, i (fr. Greek στίμμι, a blacking for eyebrows made of antimony) antimony.

ori'go, inis (f) (fr. *orior*, to rise) a rising, origin.

rete, is (n) (cogn. w. σειρά, a rope; old form *srete*) a net.

salix, i'cis (f) (kindred with *salax*, leaping, from its rapid growth) willow.

sapo, ō'nis (m) (kindred with *sebum*, grease) soap.

serpi'go, inis (f) (*serpo*, to creep) a ring-worm.

silex, Icis (m) (unknown) flint.

tabes, is (f) (fr. *tabeo*, to waste away) a wasting disease.

coxa, æ (Sansk. *kaksha*, hip) the hip point.

rectifica'tus, a, um (fr. *rectum*, right, and *facio*, to make)

reduc'tus, a, um (fr. *reduco*, to reduce) reduced.

rig'idus, a, um (fr. *rigor*, stiffness from cold) rigid.

rotun'dus, a, um ((fr. *rota*, a wheel) wheel-shaped, round.

sali'nus, a, um (fr. *sal*, salt) saline.

sanus, a, um (cognate with σαός, safe) sound, healthy.

sati'vus, ā, um (fr. *sero*, to sow) cultivated.

scale'nus, a, um (fr. Greek σκαληνός, irregular) scalene.

A. 1. Cave ne ferri sulphas admisceatur cum acido tannico. 2. Potet æger poculum aquae calidae bis in die. 3. Foveatur abscessus cum cataplasmati seminum lini. 4. Usurpet æger infusum scammonii dum eodem respondeat. 5. Misce unciam tincturae opii cum unciis tribus linimenti saponis. 6. Signa, "Admoveatur in puncto inflammationis." 7. Removeat chirurgus sequestrum ex osse. 8. Vomer et cartilago triangularis septum nasi formant. 9. In retinis occulorum spectrum formetur. 10. Adhibe emplastrum sinapis ut rubor cutis cieatur.

B. 1. The expectoration in phthisis is purulent. 2. The origin of the cranial nerves is in the brain. 3. The circular muscle of the mouth is a sphincter. 4. The pancreas is a racemose gland. 5. Salicylic acid is in the willow. 6. Apply soap liniment to the swelling. 7. Excite vesication over the hip by plaster of Spanish fly. 8. Purge the sick man with calomel and jalap. 9. Mix an ounce of tincture of aconite with five ounces of chloroform liniment. 10. Let the same stand, and mark, "To be applied on the skin."

The future past participle with *est* is often used with an imperative signification. The *est* is seldom expressed. Thus, we write, "*Fiat massa in pilulas duodecim dividenda*" (*est*), "Let there be made a mass to be divided into twelve pills."

The *ablative absolute* is sometimes used in prescription writing. Thus, "*Eodem decocto, cola et adde liquoris ammoniæ uncias duas*," "After this (same) has been boiled down, strain and add two ounces of solution of ammonia."

VERBS OF THE THIRD CONJUGATION.

	ACTIVE VOICE.		PASSIVE VOICE.		
Infinit.	Imp. 2d person sing.	Subj. 3d person sing.	Infinit.	Subjunct.	Gerund.
	add, add thou	adlat, let him add	addi, to be added	addatur, let it be added	addendus, about to be added [added
Addere, to add	adde	addat	addi	addatur	addendus
Bibere, to drink	bibe	bibat	bibi	bibatur	bibendus
Capere, to take	cape	capiat	capi	capiatur	capiendus
Colluere, to wash	colluc	colluat	collui	colluatur	colluendus
Concutere, to shake	concute	concutiat	concuti	concutiatur	concutiendus
Contundere, to bruise	contunde	contundat	contundi	contundatur	contundendus
Coquere, to cook	coque	coquat	coqui	coquatur	coquendus
Digerere, to digest	digere	digerat	digeri	digeratur	digerendus
Dividere, to divide	divide	dividat	dividi	dividatur	dividendus
Exprimere, to press out	exprime	exprimat	exprimi	exprimatur	exprimendus
Extrahere, to draw out	extrahe	extrahat	extrahi	extrahatur	extrahendus
Facere, to make	fac	faciat	fieri	fiat	faciendus
Mittere, to send	mitte	mittat	mitti	mittatur	mittendus
Ponere, to place	pone	ponat	poni	ponatur	ponendus
Solvere, to dissolve	solve	solvat	solvi	solvatur	solvendus
Sumere, take	sume	sumat	sumi	sumatur	sumendus
Terere, to rub	tere	terat	teri	teratur	terendus
Urere, to burn	ure	urat	uri	uratur	urendus
Recipere, to take	recipe	recipiat	recipi	recipiatur	recipiendus
Vomere, to vomit	vome	vomat	vomi	vomatur	vomendus

VERBS OF THE FOURTH CONJUGATION.

	ACTIVE VOICE.		PASSIVE VOICE.		
Infinit.	Imperat.	Subjunct.	Infinit.	Subjunct.	Gerund.
Deglutire, to swallow	degluti	deglutiat	deglutiri	deglutiatur	deglutiendus
Dormire, to sleep	dormi	dormiat			
Haurire, to drink	hauri	hauriat	hauriri	hauriatur	hauriendus
Partire, to divide	parti	partiat	partiri	partiatur	pariendus

VOCABULARY XXX.

talis, e, such a, such.

stramo'nium, i (fr. root *stra*, strew; cf. *strages*, slaughter) poison thornapple.

stratum, i (fr. *sterno*, to lay down) a layer.

succeda'neum, i (from *sub*, under, after, *cedo*, to follow) a substitute, successor.

suc'cinum, i (fr. *succus*, juice, supposed source) amber.

supercil'ium, i (fr. *super*, over, *cilium*, eyelash) eyebrow.

tanace'tum, i (corrupted fr. ἀθανάσια, immortality) tansy.

tig'lium, i, croton plant.

triho'rium, i (*tres*, three, and *horae*, hours) three hours.

trios'teum, i (from Greek τρίς, three, ὀστέον, bone, from form) fever root.

trit'icum, i (fr. *tero*, to thresh) wheat, dog grass.

tym'panum, i (Greek τύμπανον, a drum, from τύπτω, to strike) drum of ear.

infans, i (*in*, not, *fans*, speaking) infant.

tempus, ōris (n) (fr. root *tem*, to cut) time; the temple; the fatal spot.

tendo, ĭnis (m) (fr. *tendo* (v.) to stretch) a tendon.

testu'do, ĭnis (f) (fr. *testa*, a shell) tortoise; scalp tumor.

sciat'icus, a, um (fr. Greek ἰσχιατικός, belonging to thigh.)

sclerot'icus, a, um (from Greek σκληρός, hard) hard membrane of the eye.

serra'tus, a, um (fr. *serra*, a saw) saw-toothed, serrated.

siccus, a, um (cf. *sitio*, to be dry) dry.

sol'idus, a, um (fr. *solum*, the ground) solid.

somnif'erus, a, um (fr. *somnus*, sleep, *fero*, to bring) sleep bringing.

spu'rius, a, um (kindred with σπορά, scattering seed) illegitimate, adulterated.

sublima'tus, a, um (fr. *sublimo*, to raise up) sublimated.

surdus, a, um (fr. *sordidus*, dirty, dirt in ears) deaf.

pluvia'lis, e (fr. *pluvia*, rain) belonging to rain.

pocula'ris, e (fr. *poculum*, a cup) cup-like.

pola'ris, e (cf. Greek πόλος, a pivot) polar.

o'pium, i (Greek ὄπιον, poppy juice) opium.

pons, pontis (m) (cogn. with πάτος, a path) a bridge.

præpu'tium, i (from *præ*, before, ποσθίον, foreskin,
    first found in Satires of Juvenal) foreskin.

præscrip'tio, ŏ'nis (f) (from *præ*, before, *scribo*, to write)
    prescription.

EXERCISE XXX.

A.   1. Recipe magnesii sulphatis drachmas duas,
et pulveris glycyrrhizae drachmam unam.   2. Fiant
chartulae sex.   3. Signa, "Sumat æger unam bis in
die."   4. Urat asthmaticus folia stramonii et tabaci.
5. Oleum tanaceti est medicamentum abortifaciens.
6. Recipe florum sambuci libras duas, coque in aquae
octoriis quatuor, foveantur eodem decocto sæpius in die,
caput, facies, oculi, aliæque partes, erysipelate tentatae.
7. Oleum tiglii est catharticum drasticum.   8. Recipe
codeinae grana sex, extracti hyoscyami grana quatuor,
camphorae monobromatae grana duodecim, tere et commisce, fiat massa.   9. Eadem in pilulas decem partienda
est.   10. Signa, "Degluiat ægra unam earundem omni
bihorio donec dormiat.

B.   1. The tendon of Achilles is the strongest cord
of the body.   2. The sciatic nerve is the seat of disease.
3. The sclerotic covering of the eye is white and hard.
4. The great serrated muscle of the trunk.   5. Let the
patient (*æger*) drink an ounce of whisky.   6. Let him
swallow warm water with mustard until he vomits.
7. Take of chalk mixture and of paregoric an ounce.
8. Mix together and mark, "Shake, and let the infant
(*infans*) take a teaspoonful every three hours."   9. Put a
mustard plaster over his stomach.   10. Give him a quarter of a grain of morphine.

CHAPTER XVIII.

ADVERBS.

ADVERBS may be divided into two classes, *primitive* and *derivative*.

I. The *primitive* adverbs are few in number, and in many cases are cognate with prepositions, or with slight changes are employed as prepositions.

The following are the principal primitive adverbs:—

ante (kindred with Gk. *ἀντσα*, before) before.
cras (ety. unknown) to-morrow.
dein, thereupon.
heri (cf. *hestertus*, of yesterday, Ger. *gestern*) yesterday.
ibi (cf. *is*) there.
in'terim (cf. *inter*, between) meanwhile.
ita (cf. *ista*, that) so.
juxta (cf. *jungo*, to join) near by.
jam (cf. German *ya*) already.
nunquam (*ne*, not, *usquam*, ever) never.
nunc, (*num-ce*) now.
postea (fr. *post*, after) afterward.
quum (allied to *qui*, which) when.
satis (unknown) enough.
sic (fr. *si*, if) so.
tunc (*tum-ce*) then.
ubi (analogue of *ibi*) where.
vix (fr. root *vig*, strength) requiring strength; hardly.

II. *Derivative adverbs* are usually formed from nouns or adjectives.

1. *Adverbs are derived from nouns:*

(*a*) By adding the suffix *im* or *atim* to the stem, thus forming adverbs of manner.

Examples: From *status*, a standing point, we have *statim*, from the place where one stands, immediately; from *gradus*, a step, *gradatim*, by steps, gradually; from *gutta*, a drop, *guttatim*, by drops, drop by drop.

(*b*) The ablative case of many nouns is used adverbially. Thus we have *mane*, in the morning, (nom. wanting); *nocte*, at night, from *nox*; and *hodie*, to-day, from *hoc die*, on this day.

2. *Adverbs are derived from adjectives:*

(*a*) By adding *e* to the stem of the adjectives.

Examples: From *cautus*, careful, we have *caute*, carefully; from *jucundus*, pleasant, we have *jucunde*, pleasantly; from *plenus* full, we have *plene*, fully, from *sæpis*, frequent, we have *sæpe*, often. In a few instances the vowel of the adverbial stem differs from that of the adjective; thus we have *bene*, well, from *bonus*, an old form of *bonus*, good.

(*b*) The ablative case, masculine, of some adjectives, is used adverbially.

Examples: From *citus*, quick, we have *cito*, quickly; from *creber*, frequent, *crebro*, frequently; and from *tutus*, safe, *tuto*, safely.

VOCABULARY XXXI.

unguen'tum, i (fr. *un'gere*, to anoint) ointment.

vac uum, i (fr. *vacuus*, empty) an empty space.

velum, i (*vehulum*, fr. *ve'here*, to carry) a sail, veil.

vene'num, i (cf. Sansk. *vasha*, and Latin *virus*) poison.

vera trum, i (cf. *veratrix*, a soothsayer) soothsayers' plant, hellebore.

vinum, i (cognate with οἶνος, wine) wine.

borboryg'mus, i (fr. Greek βορβορύζω, to have a rumbling of bowels) rumbling of bowels.

pruri tus, ûs (fr. *prurio*, to itch) itching.

intro'itus, ûs (m) (fr. *intro*, within, *ire*, to go) entrance.

ulcus, cĕris (n) (cognate with Greek ἕλκος, a wound) ulcer.

varix, ĭcis (m) (fr. *varus*, stretched or bent) dilated vein.

venter, tris (m) (cognate with ἔντερον, intestine) belly.

venus, nĕris (f) (*Venus*, the goddess of love) sexual love, copper.

vertex, ĭcis (m) (fr. *verto*, to turn) the turning point, top.

verti'go, ĭnis (f) (fr. *verto*, to turn or reel) dizziness.

viscus, ĕris (n) (cf. ἴσχω, to hold) a vital organ.

vox, vocis (f) (*voco*, to call, Gk. ὄψ, voice) voice, a word.

vulnus, nĕris (n) (cf. ἕλκος, a wound) a wound.

incis'io, ō'nis (f) (*in*, into, *caedo*, to cut) incision.

porten'sis, e (fr. Portuguese city, *Oporto*) Port.

potentia'lis, e (fr. *potesse*, to be able) potential.

praten'sis, e (fr. *pratum*, a meadow) growing in meadows.

puerpera'lis, e (fr. *puer*, a boy or child) child-bed (adj.)

pyramida'lis, e (fr. πυραμίς, a pyramid) pyramidal.

radia lis, e (fr. *radius*) radial.

rena'lis, e (fr. *ren*, a kidney) renal.

renifor'mis, e (fr. *ren*, a kidney, and, *forma*, form) kidney-shaped.

semiluna'ris, e (from *semi*, half, *luna*, moon) half moon-shaped.

semina'lis, e (fr. *semen*, seed) seminal.

ses'silis, e (fr. *sedeo*, to sit) without a stem.

spina'lis, e (fr. *spina*, a thorn) spinal.

spira lis, e (fr. Greek σπεῖρα, a coil) spiral.

ster'ilis, e (Greek στερρός, hard, barren) unfruitful, barren

mons, montis (fr. root *min*, to jut) mountain, hill.

morsus, ûs (fr. *mordeo*, to bite) a biting, muzzle, grip.

diab'olus, i (fr. Gk. διαβάλλω, to scheme) schemer, devil.

A.   1. Curare tuto, cito, et jucunde, est ars medica.
2. "Ubi pus, ibi incisio," dicit chirurgus.   3. Recipe
magnesii carbonatis drachmas duas.   4. Adde gradatim
et guttatim olei cinnamomi drachmam unam.   5. Tere
bene et caute, tunc infunde aquae destillatae octarios
duos.   6. Mons Veneris et introitus vaginae sunt partes
pudendorum feminae.   7. Morsus diaboli est nomen
extremitatis fimbriatae tubi Fallopiani.   8. Ulcus per-
forans calcis morbus rarus est.   9. Jecur, lien et cap-
sulae suprarenales viscera abdominis sunt.   10. Pulsus
causatur ab actione cordis.

B.   1. The renal veins are larger than the renal
arteries.   2. The semilunar cartilages of the knee-joint.
3. The "little seminal bladders" are receptacles of the
spermatic fluid.   4. Let the sick man take a dose of
castor oil to-morrow morning.   5. A uterine tumor
without a pedicle.   6. Loss of blood causes dizziness.
7. Ointment of mercury for groin lice.   8. There is no
air in a vacuum.   9. Shake well together and let it stand
until to-morrow morning.   10. In the brain there is an
interposed veil.

CHAPTER XIX.

PREPOSITIONS.

PREPOSITIONS may be divided into three classes, according to the cases which they govern.

I. Prepositions followed by the accusative.

ad (in composition, *ac, af, al, am, ar, at*) to, toward. *Af*ferent.

ante (cogn. with ἀντί) forward, before. *Ante*flexion.

circum (Sanskrit *kakras*, a ring) around, about. *Circum*flex.

contra (English *counter-*) against, opposite. *Contra*-indication.

extra (fr. *extera*) outside of, without, beyond. *Extra*-vasation.

infra (fr. *infera*) below, beneath. *Infra*scapular.

inter (*intus*, in composition *intro*) between, among. *Inter*vascular.

per * (Greek παρά, in comp. *pel*) through. *Per*forans.

post (allied to *pono*, to place) after, behind. *Post*-humous.

præter (fr. *præ*, before) past, besides. *Preter*natural.

propter, on account of.

secundum (*secundus*) according to.

supra (fr. *super*) above, over. *Supra*scapular.

trans (Sansk. *te*, in comp, *tra*) across. *Trans*mit.

ultra (cf. *ultimus*) beyond. *Ultra*marine.

II. Prepositions governing the ablative.

a, ab or **abs** (Greek ἀπό) away, from, by. *Ab*scess.

cum (in composition *con, col, cor, cop*) with, together. *Con*cede.

---

* *Per*, in composition meaning intense or excessive, is akin to the Sanskrit *para*, much. Thus, *pertussis, perchloride*, mean, etymologically, a severe cough, a great chloride.

13

de, from, away, concerning. *De*port.

e, ex (Greek *ἐκ*) out of, out, except. *Ex*press.

præ (Greek *πρό*, in comp. *præ*, before. *Pre*fer.

pro (Greek *πρό*) before, forward. *Pro*cess.

sine (cf. *sino*, to desist) without. *Sine*cure.

III. Prepositions governing the accusative after verbs of motion and the ablative when denoting location.

in * (in comp. *il, im, ir*) into, in; *un*, against. *In*fer, *in*complete.

sub † (in comp. *suc, suf, sur, sus*) under, near, somewhat. *Sub*clavian.

subter (fr. *sub*) down under. *Subter*fuge.

super (Greek *ὑπέρ*) over, above, excessive. *Super*-foetation.

The following prepositions are used in composition only:—

amb, ambi (cf. Greek *ἀμφί*) on both sides. *Ambi*-dextrous, literally, right-handed on both sides.

di, dis (cf. Greek *διά*) apart, *un*-. *Di*vide, from *dis*, apart, *vido*, to see. *Dis*ease.

re, again, back. *Re*lapse; *re*medy, to heal again.

retro, behind. *Retro*-pharyngeal, behind the pharynx.

se (*seco*, to divide) apart. *Se*clude.

It is quite important that the student learn the exact meanings of prepositions. Although not much employed separately, they are of very frequent occurrence in the composition of medical terms.

---

* *In*, as a negative prefix, is a different word entirely from the preposition *in*. The former is akin to the Greek *ἄνευ*, without, and English *un*, while the latter is cognate with the Greek *ἐν* and *εἰς*, in and into.

† *Sub* often has the signification of English *ish*. Thus, *sub*flava, somewhat yellow, yellow*ish*. A *sub*luxation is not a luxation downward, but "somewhat of a luxation," a partial luxation or sprain.

VOCABULARY XXXII.

luxa'tio o'nis (f) (fr. *luxo*, to dislocate) dislocation.

quantus, a, um, how much; as much as.

tantus, a, um, so much.

tep idus, a, um (fr. *tepeo*, to be warm) tepid, lukewarm.

tertia'nus, a, um (fr. *tertius*, third) belonging to third day.

trigem'inus, a, um (fr. *tres*, three, *geminus*, a twin) triplet.

ustus, a, um (fr. *uro*, to burn) burnt.

varus, a, um (kindred with *verto*, to bend) bandy-legged, bow-legged.

verus, a, um (cf. German *wahr*) true, real.

semis'sis, e (fr. *semi*, half) half.

suavis, e (cogn. with ἡδύς, sweet) pleasant.

talis e (cf. *tam*, as) such.

tempora'lis, e (fr. *tempus*, temple) belonging to the temple.

therma'lis, e (fr. Gk. θέρμος, heat) pertaining to hot baths.

transversa'lis, e (*trans*, across, *verto*, to turn) transverse.

trifacia'lis, e (*tres*, three, *facies*, face) trifacial.

mediasti'num, i (*medius*, middle) middle space of thorax.

nu'bilis e (fr. *nubes*, a cloud or veil) fit to be veiled, *i. e.* marriageable.

pal'pebra, æ (fr. *palpo*, to stroke, caress) eyelid.

EXERCISE XXXII.

A. 1. Recipe tantam aquam tepidam quantam sufficit. 2. Recipe olei Ricini unciam cum semisse. 3. Nervi trigemini sunt par quintum cranii. 4. In abdomine sunt intestina magna et parva praeter organa alia. 5. Supraspinatus et infraspinatus sunt musculi scapulares. 6. Dicit Hippocrates, "Femina nunquam ambidextra est." 7. Recipe hydrargyri cum creta unciam. 8. Divide in chartulas numero viginti. 9. Liquor synovialis circum artus est. 10. In pariete

abdominis anteriore sunt musculi recti, obliqui et trans-
versales praeter musculum pyramidalem.

B.   1. The trifacial is the sensory nerve of the face
and head. 2. Also the motor nerve of the lower jaw.
3. The physician treats the patient according to art.
4. Take of saccharated pepsin three drachms and a half.
5. Divide into twelve powders. 6. Mark, "One to be
taken immediately after food. 7. Scrofula and hip-joint
disease are often (*sæpe*) tubercular. 8. Under the circular muscle of the eyelids is the "over-the-orbit" nerve.
9. The fever and the emaciation go with equal step.
10. According to law a girl is marriageable at the age of
puberty.

CHAPTER XX.

CONJUNCTIONS.

IN the following list will be found the principal conjunctions used in medical Latin.

ac, atque, and	**postquam,** after
aut, or	**quam,** than
aut—aut, either—or	**quasi** (*quam si*) as, if
autem, but	**-que,** and
donec, until	**quia,** because
dum, while	**quoad,** as long as
et, and	**quoque,** also
et—et, both—and	**sed,** but
etiam, also	**si,** if
ergo, therefore	**ut,** in order to
nec—nec, neither—nor	**-ve,** or
	vel, or

Que is attached to the latter of two words of similar construction to denote that they are co-ordinate; thus *levator labii superioris alaeque nasi,* "the lifter of both the upper lip and wing of nose. *Levator labii superioris et alae nasi,* would mean, "the lifter of the upper lip and the sides of nose."

Dum, donec, quia, quoad, and ut, are followed by the subjunctive.

VOCABULARY XXXIII.

comes, itis (m) (fr. *cum*, write, *ire*, to go) companion.
hallux or **hallex,** icis (m), the great toe.
medica′trix (id.) (adj.) (*medeor*, to cure) healing.
pes, pedis (m) (cognate with πούς, foot) foot.

pollex, īcis (m) (from *polleo*, to be strong like *Pollux*, the
wrestler) thumb or great toe.

pulvis, ĕris (m) (kind. w. *πάλη*, fine meal) dust, powder.

pulvi nar, na'ris (n) (fr. *pulvinus*, an elevation) a pillow.

stercus, ŏris (n) (cf. *tergeo*, to wipe off, cogn. with English *turd*) excrement.

tal'ipes, ĕdis (m) (fr. *talus*, ankle, *pes*, foot) club-foot.

unguis, (id.) (m) (cogn. with *ὄγκος*, a hook) a finger-nail.

valgus, a, um (cf. *ἄλγος*, pain) knock-kneed.

ventra lis, e (*venter*, belly) belonging to belly.

versic'olor (id.) (adj.) (*verso*, to change, *color*, color)
variegated.

viab'ilis, e (from French *vie*, life, able to live, or from *via*,
a road, journey) able to move, quickened.

vir'idis e (fr. *vireo*, to be green) green.

verru ca, æ (fr. *verres*, a boar) a wart or excrescence seen
on hogs.

poples, ĭtis, the ham strings.

porri'go, inis (f) (from *pro*, forth, *rego*, to extend, spread
out) dandruff, tinea capitis.

vicis (gen., no nom.) (f) (Aryan root *vik*, yield) a change,
period, time.

vica'rius, a, um (fr. *vicis*, change) substituted, exchanged.

villus, i (Aryan root *var*, to cover) shaggy hair.

EXERCISE XXXIII.

A. 1. Post hoc vel cum hoc ergo propter hoc est
argumentum medicorum.   2. "Ubi tres medici ibi duo
atheistes."   3. Vis medicatrix naturae est remedium
potentiale.   4. Pollex pedis est hallux vel digitus
maximus.   5. Arteria femoralis venas comites habet, sed
aorta earundem nullas habet.   6. Puer talipedem equi-
num habet.   7. Vomitus stercoris signum ilei est.   8. Si
herniam umbilicalem infans habeat, tunc admoveatur

emplastrum picis. 9. Vertebra prominens est septima
cervicis vertebrarum. 10. Pityriasis versicolor est morbus communis.

B. 1. In the fourth month the fœtus is viable.
2. Veratrum (green) is a poison. 3. Arsenic is an
apparent metal, so also is hydrogen. 4. There is sometimes vicarious menstruation. 5. Repeat this prescription twice (two times). 6. Knock-knee club-foot is not
so common as bow-leg club-foot. 7. The crown of
Venus was on the head of George the Third. 8. The
recurrent tibial artery. 9. Antimony or *stibium* is
poison. 10. If there is vomiting of excrement he
will die.

CHAPTER XXI.

PRESCRIPTION WRITING.

IN nearly all countries where a real science of medicine exists, Latin is the language employed in the writing of prescriptions. European practitioners are almost uniformly men of high classical training, and are able to use the language correctly, but in America the majority of medical students have had no experience whatever in Latin composition. Even in our literary colleges of late, the classics have been crowded out to make room for a score of sciences of which the student acquires a very superficial knowledge, so that the modern college graduate excels in nothing, and at the same time has lost a golden opportunity to familiarize himself with the ancient languages which are the basis of scientific nomenclature.

In the United States prescriptions are usually written in a language called by courtesy Latin, although we very much doubt whether a Cicero or Horace would ever suspect that the conglomerations of abbreviated medical terms which are sent to our drug stores were specimens of their native tongue.

A very little thought and study will enable the intelligent student to master the art of prescription writing. If he finds himself unable to do this, we would advise him to employ the English language exclusively, or better still, to give up all thoughts of becoming a physician.

In Europe, especially in medical publications, it is customary to write the entire prescription, directions to the patient included, in Latin. But there is now a ten-

dency, and we think a wise one, to write the directions
to the patient in the vernacular language. Any one who
has attempted to translate French prescriptions, in which
Latin is not used, has realized the great difficulty in
arriving at their meaning even with the aid of the best
dictionaries. The Latin names of drugs, however, are
quite uniform throughout Europe and America, and the
prescriptions found in English medical books and period-
icals can be understood in almost any country. Latin
names, moreover, are specific and exact, rendering mistakes impossible. If, for example, a physician ordered
snake root, either *Polygala senega, Aristolochia serpentaria* or *Cimicifuga racemosa* might be understood. But
the pharmacopœial terms *Serpentaria, Senega,* and *Cimicifuga* are restricted to particular preparations.

The word *prescription* is derived from the Latin
præ, before hand, and *scribere,* to write, and signifies the
written directions of a physician or surgeon for the preparation and use of a medicine or other means of cure.
A physician may prescribe change of climate or blood-
letting. When the apothecaries consulted the physicians
about their patients, prescriptions like the following were
often given:—"*Emitte sanguinis uncias sedecim saltem,
vel ad deliquium;* draw at least sixteen ounces of blood,
or until fainting is produced;" or "*Ad recidivium
præcavendum, detrahatur sanguis pro re nata;* to prevent a relapse, let blood be drawn occasionally."

A *formula,* (dim. of *forma,* a rule) is a written direction
for preparing and using a pharmaceutical remedy, being
more limited in its application than the word *prescription.*

Formulæ are of two kinds, *extemporaneous* or *magistral,* and *officinal. Magistral formulæ* are so called
because they are constructed by the physician, who is
supposed to be a master (*magister*) of his art, on the

instant, (*ex tempore*). *Officinal formulæ* are so designated because they are published in the pharmacopœias and are supposed to be kept ready for use in the apothecary shop (*officina*).

Furthermore formulæ may be either *simple* or *compound*. A *simple formula*, (*formula simplex*) contains but a single ingredient, while a *compound formula* (*formula composita*) contains two or more.

I.   The Parts of a Prescription or Formula.

1.   In this country it is usually customary to begin a prescription with *the name of the patient and the date*, although the majority of the books recommend that these be placed last or next the physician's name.

2.   *The heading.* In primitive societies the priest and the physician were one and the same man. When acting in his medical capacity no cure was ever undertaken without first invoking the assistance of the gods, a custom still in vogue among the Brahmins and Mohammedans. Prescriptions were begun with a prayer and at a later period when medicine had become distinct from theology, it was deemed sufficient to place the sign of the chief of the gods, Jupiter, (♃) at the beginning of the parchment. Whenever a metal which was supposed to be the property of any particular deity was prescribed, it was thought that the medicine would act with greater certainty and power if the symbol of the god were used instead of the name of the drug.   Thus:—

☽ the new moon, the symbol of Diana, was written for *silver*.

♀ the mirror of Venus, for *copper*.

♂ the shield and spear of Mars, for *iron*.

♄ the sickle of Saturn, for *lead*, etc.

At present the heading of a prescription is ℞, a sympol composed of the first letter of *Recipe*, *R*, and the sign of Jupiter, the king of the gods (♃). This is about the only relic in modern medicine showing that in ancient times medicine was practiced only by the priesthood, but, nevertheless, a relic quite as suggestive as the hairy point sometimes seen on the helix of the human ear, which Darwinians tell us proves that the ancestors of mankind were monkeys.

3. *The names and quantities of the ingredients.* The name of each ingredient should be in a line by itself. The ingredients should be placed in the following order: —

(*a*) The *basis*, or principal drug.

(*b*) The *auxiliary* or *adjuvant*, which is supposed to assist the action of the basis.

(*c*) The *corrective*, which removes or corrects some objectionable quality of the basis or adjuvant.

(*d*) The *vehicle*, which gives a proper form to the whole and serves as a means to convey it into the system.

After the name of each ingredient, in the same line, are placed the symbols denoting the quantities required. The following symbols and abbreviations are now used:—

C for *Congius*, a gallon.

O for *Octarius*, an *eighth* of a congius, a pint.

℥ for *uncia*, an ounce.

℈ for *drachma*, a drachm.

gr. for *granum*, or *grana*, grain or grains.

♏ for *minimum*, a minim, or $\frac{1}{60}$ of a drachm.

In prescribing fluids, *f*, for *fluidum*, is sometimes placed before the symbol designating the quantity, although this is not necessary. ℈, the sign for *scrupulum*, will be found in the books, but is now seldom used in prescriptions, all weights being expressed in ounces, drachms and grains. It will be observed that many of these symbols are mere abbreviations. The signs for ounce, drachm, and scruple, however, are modeled after those employed by the Arabic alchemists.

The number of ounces, drachms, and grains is expressed by means of the Roman letters i, ii, iii, iv, v, vi, etc., but fractions of grains and minims, with the exception of one-half, which is written *ss*, an abbreviation of *semisis*, half, are usually expressed by the Arabic numerals; thus, gr. $\frac{1}{4}$, a quarter of a grain, ℥$\frac{1}{25}$, a twenty-fifth of a minim.

With regard to the *grammatical construction* of this portion of a prescription it may be stated as a rule that the names of the ingredients in all *compound* formulæ should be put in the genitive case* after the quantities which are in the accusative case governed by *recipe.* Take for example: —

℞ Quininæ Sulphatis............ ℥j.
Extracti Gentianæ............gr. xxx.
Fiat Massa in pilulas xxx dividenda.

In *simple* formulæ, however, in which the ingredient is not weighed or measured, but counted, as is the case with pills, troches and suppositories, the name of the ingredient is put in the accusative case. Thus we may write: —℞ *Pilulas ferri compositas* xii, "take twelve compound pills of iron," not ℞ *Pilularum ferri compositarum* xii.

---

* When *q. s. ad, quantum sufficiat ad* is employed after the name of the last ingredient, the genitive is used. If, however, *ad* is used and the *q. s.* is omitted, the name of the ingredient should always be put in the accusative. Thus we may write :—*Aquæ q. s. ad unciam*, as much of water as may be needed up to an ounce, or *aquam ad unciam*, *aquam* being in the accusative governed by *recipe*, while the quantity, *unciam*, is in the accusative governed by the preposition *ad*.

It is customary with physicians to abbreviate the names of drugs used in prescriptions, partly to save time and space, but largely to cloak their ignorance of Latin grammar. When Pompey was about to consecrate a temple to Victory a dispute arose as to whether the inscription should read "*Consul Tertio*" or "*Consul Tertium*," and it was finally decided to leave the matter open for discussion by writing "*Consul Tert.*" Physicians now adopt the same plan, "when in doubt, abbreviate." But the practice is objectionable and sometimes dangerous. Pareira mentions a case in which *hydrocyanic* acid was dispensed for *hydrochloric* acid in a prescription reading *Acid hydroc. Aqua fortis* has been given for *aqua fontis*, and the abbreviation *hydr.* may mean *hydrargyrum, hydras, hydriodas, hydrochloras, hydrochloricum, hydrocyanicum*, etc. The following rules may be laid down to govern the student in writing the names of ingredients:—

(*a*) The orthography should be that which is customary.

(*b*) Abbreviations should be employed sparingly and with great caution, if at all.

(*c*) Symbols and signs should be carefully made.

(*d*) The ingredients should be designated by their pharmacopœial names.*

(*e*) Designate weights in Troy grains, ad avoirdupois ounces and pounds.

---

* The courts have decided that a physician violating this rule is guilty of contributary negligence in case the dispenser makes a serious error. If, for example, a physician prescribes *Hydrarg. Chlorid.*, intending *Hydrargyri Chloridum Mite*, and the druggist dispenses *Hydrargyri Chloridum Corrosivum*, both physician and druggist could be convicted of manslaughter if the error should cause the death of a patient.

In a file of prescriptions recently examined by the writer the following violations of this rule were observed:—*Sol. Fowler*, for *Liquor Potassii Arsenitis; Hux. Tinc.*, for *Tinctura Cinchona Composita; Chloric Ether*, for *Spiritus Chloroformi; Aq. Lima (?)* for *Liquor Calcis; Trotch. Pot.*, for *Trochisci Potassii Chloratis;* and *Pulv. Doveri*, for *Pulvis Ipecacuanha et Opii.*

In the same lot of prescriptions was one calling for calomel in an aqueous solution.

(*f*) Designate measures in minims, fluiddrachms, fluidounces, and pints, using the Roman letters instead of Arabic numerals.

4. *The directions to the compounder.* These should always be written in Latin. They declare the manner in which the prescription is to be prepared and delivered. The verbs used are in the imperative mood, as *coque misce,* boil, mix; the subjunctive present active or passive, *dividat, dividatur,* let him divide, let it be divided, or the future passive participle in *dus.* In the following sentence the three modes will be found: "*Commisce bene ut fiat massa (quæ) in pilulas duodecim dividenda (est)*; Mix well together in order that a mass may be made, which is to be divided into twelve pills."

5. *The directions to the patient.* These are preceded by the word *Signa,* or the abbreviation *Sig.,* being the imperative mood of the verb *signare,* to mark. After this should be written in English the exact method in which the patient is to use the medicine, if you would avoid the risk of having suppositories swallowed and lotions injected.

When poisonous drugs, especially those to be used externally, are prescribed, it is well to have the bottle marked "*Poison,*" but where the medicine is to be used internally, this would sometimes cause unnecessary anxiety.

In the examples of prescriptions which follow, Latin is employed in giving the directions to the patient, not that this is advisable, but that the student may become familiar with this custom, thus enabling him to understand the prescriptions found in many foreign works.

6. *The name and address of the prescriber* should be placed at the end of all prescriptions. In some countries no prescription will be compounded unless thus signed.

In order to illustrate the foregoing principles, we give the following example of a prescription: —

(1) *Address and date.*
(2) *Heading.*
(3) *Name and quan-*
    tities of ingredients.
    (*a*) *Basis.* (*b*) *Adjuvant.*

    (*c*) *Corrective.* (*d*) *Vehicle.*
(4) *Directions to compounder.*
(5) *Directions to patient.*

(6) *Name and address of pre-*
    scriber

(1) For Mrs. Sarah Jones.
    (1) January 30, 1888.
(2) ℞ (3) Liquoris Ammonii Acetatis (*a*) ℥j.
    Vini Antimonii (*b*),   ℥ivss.
    Tincturae Cardamomi Com-
      positae (*c*),   ℥j.
    Aquæ Menthæ Piperitæ (*d*) ℥iss.
(4) Fiat mistura.   Signa: (5) Cujus
    cochleare parvum in cyatho aquæ
    omni semihorio sumendum.
    (6) JOHN PHYSICK, M. D.,
      No. 18 Brown Street.

There are many terms peculiar to the language of prescriptions which are often abbreviated. In the following list the principal of these will be found: —

LATIN.	ABBREVIATION.	ENGLISH.
Absente febre	absent. febr.	fever being absent
Ad libitum	ad lib.	at pleasure
Adstante febre	adst. febr.	fever being present
Adde or addatur	add.	add
Alternis horis	altern. horis	every other hour
Ampulla, æ	ampull.	a large bottle
Ana	āā	of each
Aqua adstricta	aq. adst.	ice
Aqua bulliens	aq. bull.	boiling water
Aqua communis	aq. com.	common water
Aqua pluvialis	aq. pluv.	rain water
Bis in dies	bis in d.	twice a day
Bulliat	bull.	boil, or let it boil
Cum	c.	with
Capiat	cap.	let the patient take
Cochleare amplum vel magnum	coch. amp. vel mag.	a tablespoon.
Cochleare medium	coch. med.	a dessertspoon

LATIN.	ABBREVIATION.	ENGLISH.
Cochleare parvum	coch. parv.	a teaspoon
Compositus, a, um	comp. vel co.	compound
Collutorium, i	collut.	a mouth wash
Cortex, icis	cort.	bark or peel.
Cujus	cuj.	of which.
Cyathus, i	cyath.	a wineglass
Destillatus, a, um	dest.	distilled
Dilutus, a, um	dil.	dilute
Dimidius, i	dim.	one-half
Dividatur in partes æquales	d. in p. æq.	to be divided in equal parts
Dosis, is	d.	a dose
Ejusdem	ejusd.	of the same
Electuarium	elect.	an electuary
Enema	enem.	a clyster
Fac or fiat	f.	make
Fac pilulas duodecim	f. pil. xii.	make twelve pills
Fiat haustus	f. h.	make a draught
Fluidum	fl.	fluid
Fiat mistura	f. m.	make a mixture
Fotus, ûs	fot.	a fomentation
Frustillatim	frust.	in small pieces.
Gutta or guttæ	gtt.	a drop or drops
Gargarisma, tis (n.)	garg.	a gargle
Hora somni	h. s.	on going to bed
In dies	in d.	daily
Infusum	inf.	infusion
Julepus, i	jul.	a julep
Lagena	lagen.	bottle
Linteum	lint.	lint
Lotio	lot.	a wash
Mane primo	man. prim.	early in the morning
Manipulus, i	man.	a handful
Minimum, i	m.	a minim
Misce	M.	mix
Mistura	mist.	a mixture
Mica panis	mica pan.	a crumb of bread
Mitte	mitt.	send
More dicto	mor dict.	as directed
Nocte maneque	noct. maneque	night and morning
Numero	no.	in number
Oleum	ol.	oil

LATIN.	ABBREVIATION.	ENGLISH.
Omne hora	omn. hor.	every hour
Partes æquales	p. æq.	equal parts
Pannus linteus	pann. lint.	linen cloth
Pencillium camelinum	penc. cam.	a camel's hair pencil
Preparatus, a, um	ppt.	prepared
Post cibum	post cib.	after meals
Per fistulam vitream	per fist. vitr.	through a glass tube
Pro re nata	p. r. n.	as required
Pulvis	pulv.	a powder
Quantum sufficiat	q. s.	a sufficient quantity
Quantum vis	q. v.	as much as you choose
Quotidie	quotid.	daily
Quorum	quor.	of which
Reductum or redactum	reduct.	reduced
Scatula	scat.	a pill box
Semis or semissis	ss.	a half
Semihora	semih.	half an hour
Sesuncia	sesc.	an ounce and a half
Simul	sim.	together
Solutio	sol.	solution
Tere bene simul	t. b. sim.	rub well together
Ter in die	t. i. d.	three times a day
Tinctura	tinct. or tr.	a tincture
Triturata	trit.	triturate
Trochiscus, i	troch.	a troche
Vitellus ovi	v. o.	yolk of egg
Zingiber, is	Zz.	ginger

We may illustrate an abbreviated prescription by the following for an emulsion :—

℞ Vitell. ov.................no. ij.
Ol. Amygd. am............gtt. v.
Tere bene simul et add. grad.
Ol. Morrh................ ℥viij.
Glyc..................... ℥ij.
Ac. phos. dil............. ℥j.
Vin. Xer. q. s. ad..........Oj.
F. emuls. S. Ejus. cap. aeg. coch. mag.
t. i. d. post cib.

14

This same prescription written out in full, would be : —

> ℞ Vitellos ovorum...............numero duos.
> Olei Amygalae amaræ ....guttas quinque.
> Tere bene simul et adde gradatim.
> Olei Morrhuæ..................uncias octo.
> Glycerini....................uncias duas.
> Acidi phosphorici diluti.........unciam unam.
> Vini Xerici quantum sufficiat ad...Octarium unum.
> Fiat emulsio, Signa, " Ejusdem capiat æger cochleare magnum ter in die post cibum."

Translating the above into English, we have : —

> Take yolks of Eggs, in number two.
> Of Oil of Bitter Almond, five drops.
> Rub well together and add gradually.
> Of Cod Liver Oil, eight ounces.
> Of Glycerine, two ounces.
> Of Dilute Phosphoric Acid, one ounce.
> Of Sherry Wine, as much as will suffice to make
>   one pint
> Let there be made an emulsion, Mark " Let the
>   patient take a tablespoonful of this three times
>   a day after meals."

Powders may be prescribed in bulk, the patient to use a specified amount as directed, or the mixed powder may be put up in separate papers, *chartulæ.* For example : —

> ℞ Pulveris Opii..................ℨij.
> Zinci Acetatis.................ℨij.
> Misce. Fiat pulvis. Signa: Hujus solve drachmam in
> aquæ calidæ Octario. Injice in more dicto.
> Or,—Misce. Fiat pulvis in chartulas xviij. dividendus.
> Solve unam in aquæ calidæ Octario, etc.

" Take of Powdered Opium, two drachms.
        of Acetate of Zinc, two ounces.
Mix.   Let there be made a powder.   Mark: Dissolve a
    drachm of this in a pint of warm water.   Inject as
    directed.
Or,—Mix.   Let there be made a powder to be divided
    into eighteen parts.   Dissolve one in a pint of warm
    water," etc.

    ℞ Extracti Colocynthidis Compositi.... ℥j.
       Hydrargyri Chloridi Mitis.........gr. ij.
Fiat massa in pilulas xij. dividenda.   Capiat mane iij. et
postea ij., si alvus, horis sex, non satis dejecerit.
" Take of Compound extract of Colocynth, a drachm.
       of Calomel, twelve grains.
Let there be made a mass to be divided into twelve pills.
    Let the patient take three in the morning and two
    more if, after six hours, the bowels have not moved
    sufficiently."

In text-books it is customary to give prescriptions
for the preparation of a single dose of a medicine.
Many physicians prefer to write prescriptions in this
manner.   Thus : —

    ℞ Quininæ Sulphatis.............gr. ij.
       Extracti Euonymi.............gr. iss.
       Oleoresinæ Piperis .... ℳj
       Fac pilulam, Mitte tales no. xxiv.
Signa. : Capiat ægra harum unam ter quaterve in
    dies statim post cibum.
" Take, Of Sulphate of quinine, two grains.
       Of extract of Wahoo, a grain and a half.
       Of Oleoresin of Pepper, one minim.
Make a pill.   Send twenty four such.   Mark:
    Let the (female) patient take one of these
    three or four times a day immediately after
    meals."

N. B.—With *fiant,* the nominative case is used;
thus, *Fiant Suppositoria, pilulæ, pulveres,* etc., but the accusative case follows *fac ;* thus, *Fac pilulas, chartulas,* etc.

In prescribing plasters, it is customary to designate the dimensions by Arabic numerals. Thus:—

℞ Emplastrum Belladonnæ, 4″ x 6″.
" Take a Belladonna plaster, four by six inches in dimensions."

In this case *emplastrum* should be in the accusative case and not the genitive.

If, however, we order plaster by weight and direct the dispenser to spread it, the genitive case is used. Example:—

℞ Emplastri Picis cum Cantharide . . . . ℨj.
Extende supra Emplastrum Resinæ et admove supra nucham.
" Take a drachm of warming plaster. Spread upon resin plaster and apply over nape of neck."

PART III

THE GREEK ELEMENT IN THE LANGUAGE OF MEDICINE.

CHAPTER I.

ORTHOGRAPHY.

THE majority of the Greek words found in medical literature have been Latinized and are declined as Latin words. Greek derivatives are so much more euphonious than the compound words formed in modern languages that we find them even in German, a language which, more than any other, avoids the importation of foreign words. No one will be surprised that our Teutonic brethren prefer *pyelitis* to the cumbersome *Nierenbeckenentzuendung*. In other European countries, not even excepting Russia and Poland, Greek has become the foundation of medical terminology.

In order to understand the exact meaning of words derived from the Greek, the student should learn the signification of the original words. To accomplish this no extensive knowledge of Greek grammar is necessary. In the *first* place the alphabet, with the Roman equivalents of the letters, should be learned. *Secondly*, a knowledge of the methods by which Greek words are put in Latin and English dress is necessary, and *thirdly*, the student should commit to memory the stems of words used to designate the various parts and functions of the body, together with the signification of a number of prefixes and postfixes.

A few hours spent in the study of etymology in this manner will enable the student to learn the meaning of a host of technical expressions which would require months of study to master in any other way. In the following pages will be given the great majority of Greek derivatives in common use with the method of their formation, and the original meaning of their component parts.

The Greek alphabet consists of twenty-four letters, as follows :—

FORM.			NAME.	ROMAN EQUIVALENT.
A	*α*		Alpha	a
B	*β*	*б*	Bēta	b
Γ	*γ*		Gamma	g
Δ	*δ*		Delta	d
E	*ε*		Epsĭlon	ĕ short
Z	*ζ*		Zeta	z
H	*η*		Eta	ē long
θ	*θ*	*ϑ*	Theta	th
I	*ι*		Iōta	i
K	*χ*		Kappa	k or c
Λ	*λ*		Lambda	l
M	*μ*		Mu	m
N	*ν*		Nu	n
Ξ	*ξ*		Xi	x
O	*o*		Omĭcron	ŏ short
Π	*π*		Pi	p
P	*ρ*		Rho	r or rh
Σ	*σ*	*ς*	Sigma	s
T	*τ*		Tau	t
Υ	*υ*		Upsĭlon	u or y
Φ	*φ*		Phi	ph
X	*χ*		Chi	ch
Ψ	*ψ*		Psi	ps
Ω	*ω*		Omĕga	ō long

1. The *vowels* are α, ε, η, ι, ο, υ, ω. Of these η and ω are always long, ε and ο always short, and α, ι and υ either long or short according to position or custom, as in Latin. The quantity of these vowels remains the same when converted into Latin as may be seen by the following examples: —

Περονή, *fibula*	pĕrŏnē'us
Λίπωμα	līpō'ma
Πάρεσις	par'ĕsis
Φόσφορος	phos'phŏrus

2. The *diphthongs* with their Roman equivalents are as follows: —

Greek, αι, ει, οι, αυ, ευ, ου, υι, becoming in Roman, æ, ē or ī, œ, au, eu, ū, yi

Thus, Γλουταῖος, becomes glūtæ'us.

Νευρασθενεῖα, becomes neurastheni'a.

3. *Breathings.* Every word in Greek beginning with a vowel or with ρ, has a breathing over the initial letter, or, in the case of diphthongs, over the second letter. The *aspirate* or *rough breathing* is equivalent to the English *h*, and is written thus ('). The rough breathing is placed over all words beginning with υ or ρ. The *smooth breathing* (') is placed over initial vowels or diphthongs to denote the absence of the *h* sound. Examples: ὕδωρ, *hydor*; αἷμα, *hæma*; ρεῦμα, *rheuma*; ἀδήν, *aden*.

4. *Nasal sounds.* Gamma (γ) before γ, κ, ξ and χ has the sound of *n* in *angle* and is changed to *n* in converting Greek words with the gamma so placed, into Latin or English. For example: —

Ἀγγεῖον, becomes in Latin angi'um.

Ἀγκύλη, becomes an'kyle.

Φάρυγξ, becomes pharynx.

Ἄγχω, becomes ancho, Latin *ango*.

5. *Changes of termination.* Greek nouns ending in *ος* and *ον* are usually converted into nouns of the second declension ending in *us* and *um*. Examples: χοληδόχος, *choled'ochus;* θύμος, *thymus;* ἄντρον, *antrum.* Genitives ending in *τος* and *δος* were changed to nouns of the third declension with genitives ending in *tis* and *dis.* Examples: βρογχῖτις, βρογχίτιδος, *bronchi'tis, bronchit'idis.*

6. The *digamma* or *vau* (F). In old Homeric Greek there was another letter, the digamma, equivalent in sound to the English *v* or *w*. Thus: ᾠόν, an egg, was originally ᾠFόν, equivalent to Latin *ovum*. There is no evidence, however, that *ovum* was derived from ᾠFόν, but both came from a common word used by the Greco-Italian race before its separation.

7. *Accents.* Accents in Greek are certain marks placed over vowels, influencing their pronunciation. Just what significance they had is not definitely known. There are three accents, the acute (´), the circumflex (˜), and the grave (`). The acute accent stands on long and short syllables alike and on any of the last three syllables of a word; the circumflex accent stands only on the long syllables and only on the last two syllables of a word; the grave accent stands only on the last syllable.

CHAPTER II.

The Parts and Functions of the Body.

IN order that the student may acquire the principles of medical terminology, it will be necessary for him to commit to memory the stems of the words which designate the various parts and functions of the body. By *stem* we mean that part of a word which remains after the prefixes, suffixes and inflectional endings have been removed, or rather, the part to which these affixes are added. For example take ἄρωμα *aro'ma*, the stem is *arom*, from which we may form *aromatic*. But the *root* of a word is that essential part which contains the original meaning, and from which the word is derived. The root of *aroma* is *ar*, from an Aryan word meaning to *plough* or *cultivate*, and secondarily to *acquire* by cultivation. Thus we have in Sanskrit *aritras*, the oxen which pulled the plough, *aritram*, the plough handle, later the helm of a ship. In Greek we have ἀρόω, to plough; ἀροτήρ, a husbandman; ἄροτρον, a plough; ἄρωμα, ploughed land, secondarily the odor of ploughed land; ἄρσην, the male who did the ploughing, and many others.

In Latin there is *aro*, to plough; *arator*, a ploughman; *aratrum*, a plough; *arvum*, a cultivated field; *armentum*, an ox for ploughing; *arma*, implements for cultivating, afterwards for fighting, etc. In English the same root appears in the old verb *ear*, to cutlivate, and in *arm*, the part of the body with which we cultivate the soil.

THE PARTS AND FUNCTIONS OF THE BODY.

STEM.	GREEK.	DERIVATION.	LATIN.	ENGLISH.
Aden	ἀδήν	lit. an acorn	glandula	gland
Amygdal	ἀμυγδάλη	lit. an almond	tonsilla	tonsil
Angi	ἀγγεῖον	fr. ἄγγος, a pail	tubulus	vessel
Antibrachi	ἀντιβραχίον	fr. ἀντί against, βραχίον arm	cubitus	forearm
Antr	ἄντρον	lit. a cave, cf. ἔντεα	antrum	cavity of Highmore
Aort	ἀορτή	fr. ἀείρω, to rise up	aorta	aorta
Arteri	ἀρτηρία	fr. ἀήρ, air, τηρέω, to carry	arteria	artery
Arthr	ἄρθρον	fr. ἄρω, to join	artus	joint
Balan	βάλανος	cf. βάλλω, to cast, lit. a nut	glans penis	head of penis
Blephar	βλέφαρον	fr. βλέπω, to look	palpebra	eyelid
Brachi	βραχίον	fr. βραχύς, short	brachium	arm
Bregmat	βρέγμα	fr. βρέχω, to be moist	sinciput	top of head
Burs	βύρσα	lit. leather pouch, fr. βοῦς, an ox	bursa	bursa
Bronch	βρόγχος	lit. the throat	bronchus	bronchus
Bubon	βουβών	lit. the groin	inguen	groin
Cardi	καρδία	Sanskrit hrid	cor	heart
Carp	καρπός	Aryan root carp, to pluck	carpus	wrist
Cephal	κεφαλή	Sanskrit kapala	caput	head
Cheil or chil	χεῖλος	fr. χείω, to open	labium	lip
Cholecyst	χολεκύστις	χολή, bile; κύστις, bladder	vesica fellis	gall bladder
Chond	χόνδρος	lit. a paste of groats	cartilago	cartilage, gristle

STEM.	GREEK.	DERIVATION.	LATIN.	ENGLISH.
Cion	κιονίς	dim. of κίων, a pillar	uvula	uvula
Clitor	κλειτορίς	lit. door tender, κλείς, a key	janitrix	clitoris
Cnem	κνήμη	perhaps fr. κνῆμος, a hill	tibia, crus	shin bone, leg
Coccyg	κόκκυξ	onomatopœic, lit. a cuckoo	coccyx	coccyx
Col	κῶλον	akin to κόλον, food	colon	colon
Celi	κοιλία	fr. κοιλός, hollow	venter	belly
Colp	κόλπος	akin to κόλπος, a gulf	vagina	vagina
Core	κόρη	lit. a maiden, doll	pupilla	pupil
Cran	κρανίον	fr. κάρηνον, head	cranium	skull
Cheir or chir	χείρ	fr. αἱρέω, to grasp	manus	hand
Dactyl	δάκτυλος	fr. δείκνυμι, to point	digitus	finger
Dermat	δέρμα	cf. Sansk. dartis, leather	cutis	skin
Dacryocyst	δακρυοκύστις	fr. δάκρυον, tear, κύστις, bladder	saccus lachrymalis	lachrymal sac
Dacryosolen	δακρυοσωλήνη	fr. δάκρυον a tear, σωλήνη, tube	ductus lachrymalis	lachrymal duct
Diaphragmat	διαφράγμα	fr. διαφράσσω, to divide	diaphragma	midriff
Didym	δίδυμος	fr. δίς twice, or δύω "two, twins"	testes	testicles
Elytr	ἔλυτρον	fr. ἐλύω, to wrap	vagina	vagina
Epicrani	ἐπικρανίον	fr. ἐπί, on, κρανίον, skull	epicranium	scalp
Epidym	ἐπιδιδυμίς	fr. ἐπί, on, δίδυμος, the testicle	epididymis	epididymis
Epiplo	ἐπίπλοον	fr. ἐπί, on, πλόον, a fold	omentum	omentum
Epithel	ἐπιθήλιον	fr. ἐπί, on, θηλή, a nipple	epithelium	epithelium
Encephal	ἐγκέφαλον	fr. ἐν, in, κεφαλή, the head	cerebrum, etc.	brain

STEM.	GREEK.	DERIVATION.	LATIN.	ENGLISH.
Enter	ἔντερον	fr. ἔντος, within	intestinum	gut
Gangl	γαγγλίον	lit. a knot	ganglion	ganglion
Gastr	γαστήρ	fr. γάω, to eat	stomachus	stomach
Genei, geni	γενειον	fr. γένυς, lower jaw	mentum	chin
Geny	γένυς	kindred with γάω, to eat	mandibulum	lower jaw
Gloss	γλῶσσα	kindred with γλωχίς, a point	lingua	tongue
Glott	γλωττίς	fr. γλῶσσα, tongue	glottis	glottis
Glut	γλουτοί	fr. γλουτός, ischium	nates	buttocks
Gnath	γνάθος	fr. γνάω, to gnaw	mentum	chin
Gonat	γόνυ	Sanskrit janu	genu	knee
Gyr	γῦρος	lit. a circle	convolutio	convolution
Hæmat	αἷμα	cf. ἔαρ εἶαρ, Sanskrit asram	sanguis	blood
Hepat	ἧπαρ	Sanskrit jakrt	hepar or jecur	liver
Hist	ἱστός	lit. a loom, fr. ἵστημι, to stand	membrana	tissue
Hymen	ὑμήν	fr. ὑφαίνω, to weave	membrana	hymen, tissue
Hyster	ὑστέρμα	fr. ὕστερμος, last, lowest	uterus	womb
Ile	εἴλεον	fr. εἴλεος, twisted	ileum	ileum
In	ἴς	originally Fἴς, whence, Lat. vis	fibra	fibre
Isthm	ἰσθμός	lit. a passage, fr. εἶμα, to go	fauces	throat
Kerat	κέρας	akin to κάρα, head	cornu	cornea
Laryng	λάρυγξ	allied to λαλέω, to talk, and ἄγχω, to choke	larynx	larynx
Lapar	λαπάρα	fr. λαπαρός, soft	lumbus	loin

STEM.	GREEK.	DERIVATION.	LATIN.	ENGLISH.
Leptomening	λεπτομήνιγξ	fr. λεπτός tender, μῆνιγξ membrane	pia mater	pia mater
Lip	λίπος	Sansk. lip, fat	adeps	fat
Mast	μαστός	fr. μάσσω, to knead	mamma	breast
Mening	μῆνιγξ	connected w. ὑμήν, membrane	meninx	membrane of brain
Mesenter	μεσέντερον	μέσος middle, ἔντερον, intestine	mesenteria	mesentery
Mesodm	μεσόδμη	μέσος middle, δόμος house, in Homer a mast-box	mediastinum	mediastinum
Metr	μήτρα	fr. μήτηρ, mother	matrix	womb
My	μῦς	fr. μύω, to shut up	musculus	muscle
Myring	μύριγξ		membrana tympani	cardrum head
Myx	μύξα	fr. μύσσω, to run at the nose	mucus	mucus
Myel	μυελός	fr. μύω, to shut in	medulla	marrow
Nephr	νεφρός	cf. German niere	ren	kidney
Neur	νεῦρον	Sanskrit nauree	nervus	nerve
Nymph	νύμφη	lit. a water sprite	nympha	nymph
O(v)	ᾠόν	originally ὠϜόν, whence	ovum	egg
Odont	ὀδούς	Sanskrit danta	dens	tooth
Œsophag	οἰσοφάγος	οἴσω, to carry, φάγον, food	œsophagus	gullet
Om	ὦμος	Sanskrit aras	humerus	shoulder
Omph	ὀμφαλός	Sanskrit nablilas	umbilicus	navel
Onynch	ὄνυξ	Sanskrit nacha	unguis	nail
Oophor	ᾠοφόρον	fr. ᾠόν, egg, φέρω, to bear	ovarium	ovary
Orch	ὄρχις	lit. an olive.	testis	testicle

STEM.	GREEK.	DERIVATION.	LATIN.	ENGLISH.
Osche	ὄσχεον	fr. ἔχω, to hold, a bag	scrotum	bag
Oste	ὄστεον	Sanskrit *osthi*	os	bone
Ophthalm	ὀφθαλμός	fr. ὄπτω, to see	oculus	eye
Ot	οὖς	Aryan *ar*, to hear	auris	ear
Pachymening	παχυμήνιγξ	παχύς, thick, μῆνιγξ, membrane	dura mater	dura mater
Paranephr	παρανεφρός	παρά, side, νεφρός, kidney	capsula suprarenalis	suprarenal capsule
Parot	παρωτίς	παρά, beside, οὖς, ear	glans parotida	parotid gland
Pancreat	παγκρέας	πᾶν, all, κρέας, flesh	pancreas	sweet bread
Pecten	πεκτήν	fr. πέκω, to shear	os pubis	pubic bone
Perinæ	περίναιον	fr. περί, around, ναίως, dwelling	perineum	perineum
Peritone	περιτώναιον	fr. περί, around, τείνω, to stretch	peritoneum	peritoneum
Perone	περόνη	lit. a pin or nail	fibula	fibula
Phall	φάλλος	lit. a pillar or image of the penis carried in Bacchanalia	penis	penis
Phac	φακός	lit. a lentil	lens	crystalline lens
Phacocyst	φακοκύστις	φακός, lens, κύστις, bladder	capsula lentis	capsule of lens
Pharyng	φάρυγξ	fr. ἀράμαχυς, noise	pharynx	throat
Phleb	φλέψ	φλέω, to flow	vena	vein
Phren	φρήν	lit. mind	diaphragma	midriff
Piar	πίαρ	Sanskrit *pi*, fat	sebum	fatty oil
Pleur	πλευρόν	fr. πλευρός, side	pleuron	pleuron
Pneum	πνεῦμων	fr. πνέω, to breathe	pulmon	lung
Pod	πούς	Sanskrit *pad*	pes	foot

STEM.	GREEK.	DERIVATION.	LATIN.	ENGLISH.
Posth	ποσθή	Sanskrit pasas, penis	preputium	foreskin
Proct	πρωκτός	fr. πρό, forth, ἄγω, to drive	anus	anus or rectum
Prosop	πρόσωπον	πρός, before, ὤψ, the eyes	facies	face
Pso	ψοά	lit. the loin	psoas, lumbus	loin
Pyel	πύελος	fr. πλύνω, to wash	pelvis renis	kidney pelvis
Pylephleb	πυληφλέψ	fr. πύλη, gate, and φλέψ, vein	vena portæ	portal vein
Pylor	πυλωρός	fr. πύλη, gate, ὁρῶ, to watch	pylorus	pylorus
Rhach	ῥάχις	fr. Aryan ragh, rough	columnaspinalis	back bone
Rhin	ῥίς	cf. ῥυέω, to polish	nasus	nose
Sarc	σάρξ	fr. σαίρω, to strip	caro	flesh
Salping	σάλπιγξ	lit. trumpet, fr. σαλπίζη sea shell	tubus	Fallopian or Eustachian tube
Sialaden	σιαλαδήν	σίαλον, saliva, ἀδήν, gland	glans salivaris	salivary gland
Somat	σῶμα	fr. σάω, to keep	corpus	body
Splanchn	σπλάγχνον	allied to σπλήν, spleen	viscus	vitals
Splen	σπλήν	fr. same root as *lien*	lien or splenium	spleen
Spondyl	σπόνδυλος	lit. a spindle	vertebra	vertebra
Staphyl	σταφυλή	lit. a grape	uvula	uvula
Steat	στέαρ	fr. ἵστημι, to stand, stiff fat	adeps	stiff fat
Stomat	στόμα	Sansk. as, breath, mouth	os	mouth
Syndesm	σύνδεσμα	συν, together, δέω, to bind	ligamentum	ligament
Tenon	τένων	fr. τείνω, to stretch	tendo	tendon
Trache	τραχεῖα	fr. τραχύς, rough	trachea	wind pipe

STEM.	GREEK.	DERIVATION.	LATIN.	ENGLISH.
Trachel	τραχηλός	fr. τραχύνω, to become rough, as in animals, when angry	collum	neck
Trich	θρίξ	perhaps fr. τρίχα, triple	capillus	hair
Thorac	θώραξ	lit. a breast plate	thorax	chest
Typhl	τυφλόν	fr. τυφλός, blind	cæcum	blindgut
Ul	(Ϝ)ουλα	fr. Aryan root vol, fold	gingiva	gum
Uranisc	οὐρανίσκος	dim. of οὐρανος, sky	palatum	palate
Urach	οὐραχός	fr. οὖρον, urine, ἔχω, to hoid	urachus	urachus
Ureter	οὐρητήρ	fr. οὐρέω, to urinate	ureter	ureter
Urethr	οὐρήθρα	fr. οὖρον, urine	urethra	urethra
Zygomat	ζύγωμα	fr. ζύγος, a yoke	arcus zygomaticus	zygoma

THE FUNCTIONS AND SECRETIONS OF THE BODY.

STEM.	GREEK.	DERIVATION.	LATIN.	ENGLISH.
Æsthesis	αἴσθησις	fr. αἰσθάνομαι, to feel	sensatio	feeling
Aphrodisias	ἀφροδισίας	fr. Ἀφροδίτη, Venus	venustas	sexual desire
Bio	βίος	Sanskrit bhid	vita	life
Blenn	βλέννα	cf. βλεννόω, to drivel	mucus	mucus
Chylo	χυλός	lit. a fluid or decoction	chyle	chyle
Chymo	χυμός	fr. χέω, to pour	chyme	chyme
Chole	χολή	fr. χλόη, green	fel, bilis	gall, bile
Colostr	κολόστρον	fr. κόλον, food	colostrum	colostrum

STEM.	GREEK.	DERIVATION.	LATIN.	ENGLISH.
Copro	κοπρός	Sanskrit *capi*	fæces	excrement
Diaphoresis	διαφόρησις	διά, through, φέρω, carry	perspiratio	perspiration
Diuresis	διούρησις	διά, through, οὐρέω, to urinate	urinatio	micturition
Dipsa	δίψα	fr. πίπτω, to fall (Curtius)	sitis	thirst
Dynam	δύναμις	fr. δύναμαι, to be able	vis	strength
Emesis	ἔμεσις	fr. ἐμέω, to vomit	vomitus	puking
Galact	γάλα	cognate with Latin *lac*	lac	milk
Genesis	γένεσις	fr. γεννάω, to produce	genesis	generation
Geust	γευστία	fr. γεύω, to taste	gustatio	taste
Gone	γονή	fr. γεννάω, to beget	semen	seed
(H)idrosis	ἱδρωσις	allied to ὕδωρ, water	sudatio	sweating
Ichor	ἰχώρ	lit. the blood of the gods	serum	serum
Kinesis	κίνησις	fr. κινέω, to move	motus	movement
Lochi	λοχεία	fr. λόγος, a bed, child-bed	lochia	"shows"
Mecon	μηκώνιον	fr. μήκων, poppy juice	meconium	meconium
Men	μήνες	fr. μήν, a month	menses	monthly sickness
Mnesis	μνῆσις	fr. μνάομαι, to remember	memoria	memory
Mydriasis	μυδρίασις	cf. μυδρός, red hot, the fire test	mydriasis	dilation of pupil
Myx	μύξα	Sansk. *nukumi*, to cast off	mucus	snot
Œstrus	οἶστρος	lit. a gad-fly, mad desire	œstrus	rutting
Orexia	ὄρεξις	fr. ὀρέγω, to desire	fames	appetite
Orgasm	ὀργησμα	fr. ὀργάω, to swell	orgasma	orgasm

15

STEM.	GREEK.	DERIVATION.	LATIN.	ENGLISH.
Osmosis	ὠσμωσις	fr. ὠσμὸς, impulse	osmosis	osmosis
Opsia	ὠψια	fr. ὄπτω, to see	visus	sight
Osphresis	ὀσφρησις	fr. ὀσφραίνομαι, to smell	olfactio	olfaction
Pareunia	παρευνια	fr. παρευνέω, to go to bed with	coitus	sexual intercourse
Phagia	φαγια	fr. φάγω, to eat	deglutio	eating, swallowing
Phasia	φασια	fr. φημί, to speak	dictio	speaking
Phemia	φημια	fr. φημί, to speak	vocatio	speaking
Phonia	φωνια	fr. φωνή, voice	vox	voice
Physis	φυσις	fr. φύω, to grow	natura	nature, growth
Pnœa	πνοια	fr. πνέω, to breathe	respiratio	breathing
Posis	ποσις	fr. πίνω, to drink	sitis	thirst
Ptysis	πτυσις	fr. πτύω, to spit	salivatio	spitting
Smegma	σμεγμα	lit. soap, cf. smago and Eng. smear	smegma	smegma
Spermat	σπέρμα	fr. σπείρω, to sow	semen	seed
Sphyxia	σφύξις	fr. σφύζω, to throb	pulsus	pulse
Uro	ουρον	Sanskrit vari	urina	urine

CHAPTER III.

PREFIXES.

THE prefixes used in Greek are prepositions, adjectives, and adverbs, or words derived from these.

a-, an-, or am- (Greek ἀ, ἀμ, or ἀν). *A-* before a *consonant*, except a few words beginning with *bl* or *br;* *an-* before a *vowel*, and *am-* before words beginning with *bl* or *br*. These are inseparable particles kindred with ἄνευ, without, and equivalent to the Latin prefix *in*, negative, and the English *un-*, as seen in *in*firm, not strong, *un*well, not well. This prefix is called *alpha privative*, and is used to form compound words denoting the absence of the thing designated by the original word, as may be seen in the following list: —

abrach'ia, without arms, armless monstrosity.
abu'lia, loss of will power, βουλή.
acar'dia (a monstrosity) without a heart.
acephal'ic, without a head, headless.
aceph'alocyst, a headless monstrosity with cyst of cord.
achei'rous, without hands, handless.
acra'nia, monstrosity without a skull.
acye'sis, inability to become pregnant, sterility.
adac'rya, non-secretion of tears.
adyna'mia, want of strength, loss of power.
agalac'tia, absence of milk in breast after delivery.
agera'sia, without old age, a green old age.
ageus'tia, loss of sense of taste.
aglos'sia, absence of tongue.
alex'ia, inability to read resulting from disease.
ambro'sia, immortality, the food of the immortals.
am'blosis, not living, abortion.

amenorrhœ'a, absence of menses.

amne'sia, loss of memory.

amor'phism, without definite form, formlessness.

anæ'mia, lit. bloodless, deficiency of blood corpuscles.

anæsthe'sia, loss of sensation.

analge'sia, without sense of pain.

anaphrodis'ia, without sexual desire.

anhy'drous, without water.

anidro'sis, suppression of perspiration.

an'odyne, without pain, a medicine curing pain.

anor'chous, without testicles.

anorex'ia, loss of appetite.

anos'mia, loss of sense of smell.

ap'athy, without mental feeling.

apep'sia, loss of digestive power.

apha'cia, absence of crystalline lens.

apha'sia, loss of speech, of memory of words.

aphe'mia, loss of speech.

apho'nia, loss of voice.

apnœ'a, cessation of breathing.

apo'sia, without thirst.

aproc'tia, without an anus.

ap'terous, wingless.

apyrex'ia, absence of fever.

asa'phia, loss of clearness of voice, hoarseness, fr. σαφής, clear.

asper'mia, non-secretion of semen.

asphyx'ia, lit. pulselessness, suffocation.

astig'matism, without a point of convergence.

asys'tole, non-contraction.

atax'ia, want of co-ordination.

atom, lit. uncut, too small to be cut.

at'ony, loss of tone, strength.

at'rophy, cessation of growth.

amphi- (ἀμφί) before consonants, *amph* (ἀμφ') before vowels. A preposition equivalent to the Latin *ambi* or *amb*, meaning literally *on both sides*, with a secondary meaning of *both ways*.

amphiarthro'sis, articulating both ways, *i. e.* synarthrosis and diarthrosis.

amphib'ious, living both ways, *i. e.* on land and in water.

am phora, handles, φόροι, on both sides, two-handled jar.

ana-, (ἀνά-) before consonants, *an-* (ἀν') before vowels. A preposition meaning *up*, *throughout*, *again*, Latin *re*, or *apart*, like Latin *se* and *dis*.

anal'ysis, a loosening again, solution.

anasar'ca, (water) throughout the flesh.

anastomo'sis, inosculation.

an'aplasty, a forming again, restoration of lost parts.

anaspa'dias, opening (σπαδία) upwards of urethra.

anode, the upward track (ὁδός) of electric current.

anti- (ἀντί-) before a vowel, *ant-* (ἀντ') before a consonant, *anth-* (ἀνθ'-) before the aspirate *h*. A preposition meaning *against*, *opposite*, *opposed to*, like Latin *contra* and English *counter*. It is often used in the formation of words denoting remedies for the affection specified by the primitive.

antephial'tes, a remedy for nightmare.

anthe'lix, (the part of ear) opposite the helix.

anthelmin'tic, a remedy for removing worms, ἕλμινς.

an'ticheir, opposite the hand, *i. e.* the thumb.

ant'idote, a counteracting medicine, given (δότος) against.

antilith'ic, a remedy for stone, *calculus*, λίθος, or for lithæmia.

antip'athy, a feeling (πάθος) against.

antiphlogis'tic, a remedy for inflammation, φλογώσις.

antipyret'ic, a remedy for fever, πῦρ.
antisep'tic, opposing putrefaction, σῆπσις.
antispasmod'ic, a remedy for spasm, σπάσμος.
antith'enar, opposite the hollow part of hand, θέναρ.
antit'ragus, opposite the tragus.

apo- (ἀπό) before consonants, ap- (ἀπ') before vowels
and aph- (ἀφ') before the aspirate h.   A preposition
meaning *away, from*, like Latin *ab*, English *off*.
aph'orism, a marking off, definition, fr. ὁρίζω, to bound.
aponeuro'sis, (expansion) from a tendon, νεῦρον.
apoph'ysis, a natural growth, φύσις, from a bone.
ap oplexy, a striking off, from πληγή, a stroke.
apoth'ecary, one who stores away drugs, from θήκη, a
storehouse.
aposte'ma, a standing away, abscess, ἵστημι, to stand.

auto- (αὐτο-) before consonants, aut- (αὐτ') before
vowels, from αὐτός, self, a reflexive pronoun.
autoplas'tic, formed from one's self, *i. e.* by taking tissue
from the patient.
au'topsy, a seeing, ὄψις, or examination of the body itself.

cata- (ἀκατ) before consonants, cat- (κατ') cath- (καθ')
before the aspirate h.   A preposition meaning *down*,
through, with a secondary meaning of *concealed*, like the
Latin *de*.
cat'alepsy, seizing upon, fr. καταλαμβάνω, to pounce upon.
catal'ysis, a *di*ssolution, or *concealed* solution.
catame nia, the monthly flowing *down* menses.
cat aplasm, something layed down, a poultice.
cat'aract, rushing down, ῥήγνυμι, to rush, opacity of lens.
cathar'tic, fr. καθαίρω, to carry down, a purgative
medicine.

cath'eter, the instrument sent down to the bladder, fr. καθίημι, to send down.

dia- (διά) a preposition allied to δύω, two, like Latin *di-* or *dis-*, apart. The meaning is *through*, like Latin *per*.

diabe'tes, a running through, fr. διαβαίνω, to go through.

diachy'lon, a plaster made through, *i. e.* by means of juice, χυλός.

diagno sis, a knowing through, *i. e.* thoroughly, of a disease.

diapede'sis, a leaping through; (passage of blood corpuscles through wall of vessel).

diaph'anous, shining through, transparent.

diaph'ysis, a growing through or between; the shaft of a bone.

di'astase, the substance which dissolves, fr. δια-ίστημι, to separate.

dias'tole, a sending apart, dilatation, from διαστέλλω, to dilate.

diath'esis, a placing through, constitution, διατίθημι, to arrange.

diet, a regulation, regimen, fr. διαιτέω, to regulate.

dys (δύς) an inseparable adverbial prefix like the Sanskrit *dus* and English *mis*. The meaning is *bad*, *difficult*, *painful*, or *defective*.

dyscra'sia, bad temperament, κρᾶσις.

dyseco'ia, defective hearing, ἀκοή.

dys'entery, lit. a difficulty with the bowels, inflammation of colon.

dysla'lia, slow difficult speech, λαλία.

dyslex'ia, pain in eyes caused by reading.

dysmenorrhœ'a, painful menstruation.

dyskine'sis, painful motion or movement, κίνησις.

dyspareu'nia, painful sexual intercourse.

dyspep'sia, difficult or defective digestion.

dyspha'gia, painful mastication and swallowing.

dyspho'nia, defective voice, hoarseness.

dyspnœ'a, difficult respiration.

ec- (ἐκ) before a consonant, **ex-** (ἐξ) before a vowel. A preposition cognate with Latin *e* or *ex*, meaning *out, out from;* whence we have *ecto-* (ἐκτός), *outside.*

ecbol'ic, a medicine which casts out, causes abortion, from βάλλω, to throw.

eccoprot'ic, a medicine to remove fæces, κόπρος.

eccye'sis, extra-uterine pregnancy, κύησις.

eclamp'sia, an effulgence, a symptom in some convulsive diseases.

ec'phlysis, a bubbling out, vesicular eruption, ἐκφλύω, to bubble.

ecphy'ma, an outward growth, φύμα, a wart, excrescence.

ec'stasy, a standing, στάσις, out, out of one's mind.

ecthy'ma, a breaking out, pustular eruption, ἐκθύω, to break out.

ecto'pia, a displacement, τόπος, a place.

ectozo'a, external, ἐκτός, parasites or animals, ζῶα.

ectro'pion, a turning (τρέπω, to turn) out of the eyelids.

ec'zema, a boiling (ζέω, to boil) out of the humors, an eruptive skin disease, salt rheum.

exanthe'ma, a blossoming out, ἄνθημα, eruptive fever.

exog'enous, produced abroad or without, fr. γεννάω, to produce.

exom'phalus, lit. out of the navel, ὀμφαλός, umbilical hernia.

exophthal'mia, protrusion of eyeballs.

exosmo'sis, the impulse of fluids outward.

exosto'sis, an abnormal growth of bone outward.

exot'ic, foreign, ἐξότερος.

en- (ἐν), before *p* and *b*, **em-** (ἐμ). A preposition equivalent to the Latin *in* with the ablative, meaning *in, within.*

em bolism, lit. something thrown in, an arterial plug, fr. βάλλω, to throw.

emphy'ma, a growth within, subcutaneous tumor (φύμα).

emphyse'ma, an abnormal inflation with air, fr. ἐμφυσάω, to blow in.

empye ma, pus (πύον) within (pleural cavity).

empy'ocele, a scrotal tumor containing pus.

enarthro'sis, articulation in, *i. e.* ball and socket joint.

encan this, aan excrescence in *canthus* of eye.

endem'ic, a disease within a limited population, δῆμος.

ender'mic, in the skin.

en'ema, an injection, from ἐνίημι, to send in.

entro'pion, a turning in of the eyelids, from ἐντρέπω, to turn in.

errhine, lit. in the nose, a snuff.

endo- (ἐνδο) and **ento-** (ἐντο), from ἐνδος and ἐντός, within. These are adverbial expressions derived from ἐν, in, and are equivalent to the Latin *intra* and *intro.*

endan'gium, membrane lining inside of vessels.

endarte'rium, membrane lining inside of arteries.

endocar'dium, membrane lining inside of heart.

endome'trium, membrane lining inside of womb.

en doblast, inner membrane of embryo, βλάστημα, a bud.

en'doscope, an instrument for looking into cavities, σκοπέω, to look.

endosmo sis, impulse of liquids inward.

endos'teum, inner or medullary membrane of bones.

ento'phyte, a plant φυτόν growing within the body.

entozo on, a animal parasite within the body.

epi- (ἐπί) before consonants, **ep'-** (ἐπ') before vowels, and **eph-** (ἐφ) before the aspirate *h.* A preposition meaning *upon, on, over, upper.*

epen'dyma, lit. upper clothing (ἐνδυμα) lining of ventricles of brain.

epicon dyle, a tuberosity in the condyle κόνδυλος.

ephe'lis, lit. on the nail, ἧλος, a freckle.

ephem'era, for a day (ἡμέρα) a transitory fever.

ephial'tes, a leaping upon; nightmare fr. ἐφάλλομαι, to leap upon.

epican thus, on the canthus, a fold in corner of eye.

epider mis, upper skin, outer coat of skin.

epigas'trium, over-the-stomach (region).

epiglot tis, (organ) over the glottis.

ep'ilepsy, a seizing upon, fr. λαμβάνω, to seize.

epiph'ora, a carrying (φόρος) over, running over of tears.

epiph'ysis, a upper growth (of bone).

epispa'dias, opening of urethra upward.

epispas'tic, a medicine to draw (σπάω) up (a blister).

epistax'is, a distilling (στάξις) up, nose bleed.

epidem'ic, (a disease) upon the whole people (δῆμος).

epizoot'ic, a disease upon a whole specis of animals (ζῶα).

epu lis, (a tumor) on the gums οὖλα.

eu- (εὖ) an adverb opposed to *dys-* (δυς) in meaning, like Latin *bene, well, easy.*

eucalyp'tus, lit. well covered, fr. καλύπτω, to cover, blue gum tree.

euon'ymus, lit. well named, fr. ὄνυμα, the plant *Wahoo.*

eupnœ a, easy respiration.

euthana'sia, easy death (θάνατος).

euthym ia, easy frame of mind (θυμός).

hemi- (ἡμι) fr. ἥμισυς a numeral adjective meaning *half,* equivalent to Latin *semi.*

hemianæsthe'sia, loss of sensation on one side.

hemianop'sia, loss of vision in half of each eye.

hemichore'a, chorea affecting one side.

hemicra nia, (neuralgia) of half the head, megrim.

hemio pia, a disorder of vision in which but half an object is seen.

hemiple'gia, a paralytic stroke of half the body.

hem'isphere, half a sphere (σφαῖρα) half of cerebrum.

hyper- (ὑπέρ) a preposition meaning *over, above, excess of,* like the Latin *super.*

hyperidro'sis, excessive sweating.

hyperino'sis, excess of fibrin in the blood, fr. ἴς, fibre.

hyperæsthe sia, excessive feeling, or irritability.

hypercar'dia, enlargement of heart.

hyperpla sia, excessive formation of tissue.

hyperpnœ'a, rapid respiration.

hyper'trophy, excessive growth of a part.

hypo- (ὑπό) before consonants, **hyp-** (ὑπ) before vowels, and **hyph-** (ὑφ) before the aspirate *h.* A preposition meaning *below, under, deficient,* like the Latin *sub* and *subter.*

hypino'sis, deficiency of fibrin in blood.

hypochon'drium, region below the cartilages of ribs.

hypocra'nium, collection of pus under cranium.

hypoder'mic, under the skin, subcutaneous.

hypogas'trium, region below stomach.

hypoglos'sal, under the tongue, sublingual.

hypoglot tis, lower part of glottis.

hypospa'dias, opening of urethra under penis.

hypostat'ic, lit. standing under. Gravitation of blood from defective circulation.

meta- (μετά) before consonants, **met-** (μετ') before vowels, and **meth-** (μεθ') before the aspirate *h*. A preposition kindred with the Sanskrit *mithu*, together, German *mit*, and English *with* and *amidst*. A secondary meaning is *from one place to another* and *after*.

metab'olism, casting or changing about, from μεταβάλλω, to exchange.

metacar'pus, part of hand next to the carpus.

metam'erism, a change in the arrangements of the parts (μέρος) or atoms of a chemical compound.

metamor'phosis, a change of form (μορφή).

metas'tasis, a change of position, from μεθίστημι, to transpose.

metatar'sus, part of foot next to the ankle, ταρσός.

metopan'trum, the cavity (ἄντρον) between the eyes, frontal sinus.

pan- (πᾶν), **pant-** (παντ') an adjective meaning *all*, *every*, like the Latin *omnis*.

panace'a, a cure-all, from ἀκέομαι, to cure.

pandem'ic, a disease common to all people, δῆμος.

pantopho'bia, fear of all things, a symptom in some forms of insanity.

pantatro'phia, complete atrophy, as seen in dwarfs.

para- (παρά) before consonants, **par-** (παρ') before vowels. A preposition kindred with Sanskrit *para*, back, and Latin *per*, through. The original meaning was, *by the side of*, with secondary meanings of *by*, *near*, *wrong*, *abnormal*, *through*.

paracente'sis, a piercing through, fr. κεντέω, to bore.

paræesthe'sia, abnormal sensation.

paral'ysis, a loosening at the side or an abnormal relaxing of muscles.

parame'nia, abnormal menstruation, vicarious menstruation.

parame'trium, parts near the womb, tissues of pelvis.

paraphimo'sis, a muzzling φίμωσις, back of the glans penis.

paraplas'tic, abnormal formation of tissue.

paraple'gia, an abnormal stroke, *i. e.* of lower half of body.

par'asite, one who lives on the food (σῖτος) of another.

paraspa'dias, opening of urethra on side of penis.

parasys'tole, abnormal contraction of heart.

paregor'ic, soothing, fr. παραγορέω, to encourage, urge on, coach.

paratrip'tic, rubbing together, increasing waste.

paren'chyma, that which is poured in by the side of; the substance of an organ, fr ἐγχύω, to pour in.

par'esis, an abnormal ataxic movement, παρίημι, to misdirect.

paronych'ia, disease near the nail (ὄνυξ); whitlow.

parot'id, by the side of the ear (οὖς) præ-auricular.

paros'mia, perverted sense of smell (ὀσμή).

par'oxysm, an unusual sharpening, *i. e.* exacerbation, fr. ὀξύνω, to sharpen.

paru'lis, (a boil) on side of gum (οὖλα).

peri- (περί). A preposition cognate with Sanskrit *pari*, around, and Latin adverb *per* intensive, as seen in *pertussis*. Meaning *about, around,* like Latin *circum.*

periarthri'tis, inflammation of parts around a joint.

pericar'dium, the sac surrounding heart.

perichon'drium, the membrane surrounding cartilages.

pericra'nium, the membrane covering skull.

perides'mium, the membrane covering ligaments.

perridid'ymis, the serous covering of the testicle.

periglot'tis, the membrane covering tongue.
perime'trium, the serous covering of womb.
perimys'ium, the membrane covering muscles.
perineu'rium, the membrane covering a nerve.
perine'phrium, the covering (capsule) of kidney.
perios'teum, the membrane covering bones.
periph'acus, the capsule of the crystalline lens.
peripneumo'nia, inflammation around the air passages.
peristal'sis, a sending (στέλλω, to send) around, vermi-
cular motion.
peritone'um, the membrane stretched (τείνω) around
bowels.
perityph'lium, the serous covering of cæcum.

poly- (πολυ) from πολύς, many, equivalent to Latin
multus.
polycys'tic, composed of many cysts.
polydac'tylism, having supernumerary fingers.
polydip'sia, excessive thirst, δίψα.
polyphar'macy, use of many drugs (φάρμακον).
pol'ypus, having many feet or prolongations; a soft tumor.
polyu'ria, excessive secretion of urine.

pro- (πρό). A preposition equivalent to the Latin
pro and *præ*, *before*, *forward*.
prodrome, running (δρόμα) before, preliminary symptom.
proglot'tis, lit. a fore-tongue, a segment of a tape-worm
which resembles a tongue.
prognath'ic, having a projecting lower jaw, γνάθος.
progno'sis, a knowing beforehand the termination of a
disease.
prophylax'is, guarding (φυλάξις) beforehand, prevention.
prostate, the gland which stands before the bladder, fr.
προστάτης, a president or bishop.

pros- (πρός) cognate with Sanskrit *prate*, against. A preposition meaning *to*, equivalent to Latin *ad*, as in *adverse*.

prosthet'ic, adding, replacing, fr. προστίθημι, to add to. That branch of surgery which relates to restoration or substitution of lost parts, as the making of artificial teeth and limbs.

sym- (σομ), syn- (σύν), syl- (σύλ), sy- (συ), from σύν, a preposition meaning *with*, *together*, cognate with Latin *cum*, Germ. *zusamen*, and English *same*.

symbleph'aron, adhesion of eyelids.

symbol, lit. cast together, fr. βάλλω, to throw, a sign.

sym'metry, a measuring (μέτρον) together, alike.

sym'pathy, a feeling with, fellow-feeling.

symptom, falling together, fr. πίπτω, to fall, concadence.

sym'physis, a growing (φύσις) together.

syn'chronous, happening at the same time.

syn'chysis, a pouring (χύσις) together of humors of eye.

syn'cope, a cutting short of vitality, fainting, from κόπτω, to cut.

synechi'a, a holding together, adhesion of iris to cornea, from ἔχω, to hold.

syno'via, lit. white of egg (ὠFόν), fluid of joints.

syn'thesis, a putting together; composition, fr. συντίθημι, to put together.

syn'tonin, the substance which holds fibres together, τείνω, to stretch.

system, a placing together, arrangement, fr. συνίστημι, to arrange.

sys'tole, a sending together, contraction, fr. στέλλω, to send.

CHAPTER IV.

NUMERAL ADJECTIVES USED AS PREFIXES.

STEM.	GREEK.	LATIN.	ENGLISH.
Prot	πρῶτος	primus	first
Mon	μόνος	singulus	single
Di	δίς	bis or bin	twice, double
Deutero	δεύτερος	secundus	second
Tri	τρεῖς	tres	three
Tetr(a)	τέτταρες	quatuor	four
Pent	πέντε	quinque	five
Hex	ἕξ	sex	six
Hept(a)	ἑπτά	septem	seven
Oct(o)	ὀκτώ	octo	eight
Enne	ἐννέα	novem	nine
Dec(a)	δέκα	decem	ten
Hecat(o)	ἑκατόν	centum	hundred
Kilo	χίλιοι	mille	thousand
Myri(a)	μύριοι	decem millia	ten thousand

pro'teid, a first or original compound in an organism.

pro'toplasm, the first formative substance, πλάσμα.

protox'ide, the first or lower oxide.

protozo'a, the first, or lowest animals.

pro'toplast, a primary formation, fr. πλάσσω, to form.

monad, a unit, ultimate atom, combining with a single atom.

monan'drous, a plant with one stamen (ἀνήρ, a man).

monoba'sic, having a single base.

mon ograph, a writing (γραφή) on a single subject.

monoma'nia, mania with a single delusion.

monor'chis, a male with but one testicle.

di'atom, lit. an organism composed of two atoms, lowest living organism.

dichot'omous, cut in twain (δίχα), dividing by twos.

dicrot'ic, a double stroke (κρότος) of pulse.

digas tric, double bellied, Latin *biventer.*

dimor phism, having two distinct forms (μορφή).

dip loe, a doubling, fold; πλόω, to fold; two layers of cranial bones.

diplo'ma, lit. a folded parchment.

dis toma, an animal having two mouths; fluke worm.

disto'cia, birth of twins.

deuterop'athy, a *secondary* affection.

triad, an element capable of combining with three monad atoms.

trichot'omous, a dividing (τομή) by threes, τρίχα.

trisplanch'nic, belonging to viscera (σπλάγχνα) of three cavities; sympathetic nerve.

tetrad, an element capable of combining with four monad atoms.

tetran'drous, having four stamens.

pentad, an element capable of uniting with five monad atoms.

decan'drous, having ten stamens.

16

CHAPTER V.

Suffixes or Postfixes.

SUFFIXES are of two kinds: *first, inflectional* or *inseparable*, those which cannot exist separately and are employed exclusively to change the form and meaning of stems; and *secondly, separable*, those which are capable of being used alone without any connection with another word. For example, the *ness* in cold*ness* belongs to the former variety of suffixes, while the *man* of cart-*man* belongs to the latter.

1. -**æmia** or -**hæmia**, from αἷμα, blood, is used to form compound words denoting that the substance indicated by the original word is in the blood, or describes the character of the blood; the first member of the compound thus having the signification of an adjective.

acetonæ′mia, acetone in the blood.

cholæ′mia, bile in the blood.

cholesteræ′mia, cholesterin in the blood.

galactæ′mia, milk in the blood.

hyperinæ′mia, excess of fibrin in blood.

hypinæ′mia, deficiency of fibrin in blood.

hydræ′mia, watery blood.

ischæ′mia, deficiency of blood.

leucæ′mia,* excess of white blood corpuscles, fr. λευκός, white.

leucocythæ′mia, excess of white blood corpuscles, from λευκοκύτος, a white blood corpuscle.

lithæ′mia, lithic acid in the blood.

---

* Leucæmia, septicæmia and uricæmia would be more properly spelled *leuchæmia, septichæmia* and *urichæmia*, thus preserving the aspirate *h*. K should not be used for *ch* in these words.

melanæ'mia, lit. black (μέλας) blood, pigment in blood.
olighæ'mia, deficiency of blood corpuscles, ὀλίγος, few.
piarræ'mia, fat in the blood.
pyæ'mia, pus (πύον) in the blood.
sapræ'mia, putrid (matter) in blood, fr. σαπρός, rotten.
septicæ'mia, putrid blood, fr. σηπτός, putrid.
toxæ'mia, poison (τοξικόν) in blood.
uræ'mia, urea or urine in blood, fr. οὖρον, urine.
uricæ'mia, uric acid in blood.

2. -agogue. Greek ἀγωγά fr. ἄγω to lead, force, carry off. This suffix is attached to the stems of words denoting secretions or excretions, to form words signifying a remedy which will stimulate or carry them off.

chol agogue, a remedy to carry off bile.
cop ragogue, a remedy to carry off fæces.
emmen'agogue, a remedy to stimulate menstrual flow.
galact'agogue, a remedy to stimulate secretion of milk.
hy'dragogue, a remedy to carry off water from the system.
panchym agogue, a remedy to stimulate secretion of all digestive ferments.
sial'agogue, a remedy to stimulate salivary secretion.

3. -agra. Greek ἄγρα a seizure, fr. ἀγράω to pounce upon. This suffix denotes a sudden attack of pain, usually with inflammation of a gouty or rheumatic character. It is attached to the stems of words designating the part of the body affected. Ἄγρα was first employed in this manner by Aristotle.

arth'ragra, gout or rheumatism of a joint.
cephal'agra, sudden attack of pain in the head.
car'pagra, sudden attack of pain in wrist.
cheir agra, sudden rheumatic attack of hands.
cardi'agra, sudden pain in region of heart.

dactyl'agra, attack of gout or rheumatism in fingers.
gon'agra, attack of gout or rheumatism in knee.
om'agra, attack of gout or rheumatism in shoulder.
odont'agra, gouty or rheumatic toothache.
ophthal magra. gouty or rheumatic pain in eye.
pel'lagra, lit. a skin attack, Italian leprosy.
pod'agra, a gouty attack of foot, gout.

4. **-algia.** Greek ἀλγία, fr. ἄλγος pain, ache. This suffix denotes an aching or neuralgic condition of the part designated by the primitive. *Ἄλγος* in Greek differs from ὀδύνη from which *odynia* is derived in being more general in its application, and was applied to both mental and physical pain. In medicine *algia* denotes a pain of longer duration than one designated by *odynia*, although these suffixes are in many cases used synonymously.

antral'gia, neuralgia of the antrum Highmori.
arthral'gia, chronic pain in a joint.
brachial'gia, armache.
cardial gia, lit. pain in heart, now applied to pain at cardiac end of stomach.
cephalal'gia, headache.
clitoral'gia, pain in clitoris.
cœlial gia, belly ache.
cystal'gia, neuralgic pain in bladder.
dermatal gia, neuralgia of skin.
enteral'gia, pain in intestines.
gastral'gia, stomach ache.
glossal'gia, neuralgia of tongue.
hepatal'gia, pain in region of liver.
hysteral'gia, pain in womb.
mastal'gia, pain in breast.
metral'gia, pain in womb.
myal'gia, pain in muscles, muscular rheumatism.

nephral'gia, pain in region of kidney.

neural'gia, pain in a nerve.

nostal'gia, a painful longing to return home (νοστός, a return).

odontal'gia, toothache.

oophoral'gia, neuralgia of ovary.

orchial'gia, neuralgia of testicle.

ostal'gia, pain in a bone.

otal'gia, earache.

pancreatalgia, pain in region of pancreas.

phallal'gia, pain in penis.

pleural'gia, side ache.

proctal gia, pain in anus or rectum.

prosopal'gia, facial neuralgia.

rhachal'gia, backache, pain in spine.

rhinal'gia, pain in nose.

splenal'gia, pain in region of spleen.

spondylal'gia, pain in a vertebra.

urethral'gia, pain in urethra.

With the great majority of the above words, the expression "neuralgia" of the part affected may be employed synonymously.

5. **-atre'sia.** Greek ἀτρησία, from ἀ, privative, and τράω, to bore, unbored, equivalent to the Latin *imperforatio*. This suffix is attached to the stems of words designating organs of a tubular character and denotes an imperforate condition of these organs.

colpatre'sia, imperforate vagina.

enteratre'sia, imperforate intestine.

gynatre sia, imperforate condition of female (γύνη) genitals.

proctatre'sia, imperforate anus.

urethratre'sia, imperforate urethra.

6. **-ca ce.** Greek κάκη, evil, from κακός, bad. This
suffix was formerly much used to denote an ulcerated or
offensive condition of the part designated by the primitive word. The word *evil*, as employed in *poll evil*, an
ulceration on the back of the neck (*poll*) of horses, is the
exact counterpart of the Greek κάκη as a suffix. *King's
evil, scrofula,* is an ulcerous condition of the glands of
the neck, and was so called because the royal touch was
supposed to cure it.

arthroc′ace, ulcerous disease of a joint.

gonoc′ace, ulcerous condition of knee, white swelling.

rhinoc′ace, fetid ulceration of nose.

stomatoc′ace, fetid ulceration of mouth.

7. **-cele.** Greek κήλη, a *hernia, rupture.* This
suffix denotes the protrusion of an organ or part from its
normal position. It is attached sometimes to the stem
of the word designating the part protruding, and sometimes to the stem of the word designating the locality in
which the hernia exists.

bubon′ocele,* inguinal hernia, fr. βουβών, the groin.

bron′chocele, lit. a protrusion of the wind pipe, now
applied to *goitre.*

col′pocele, vaginal hernia.

cyst′ocele, hernia of the bladder.

epi′plocele, hernia of the omentum.

enceph′alocele, hernia of the brain, (ἐγκέφαλον).

en′terocele, a protrusion of the intestine.

gas′trocele, a protrusion of the stomach.

hæmat′ocele, a protruding tumor filled with blood.

hepat′ocele, a hernia of the liver or in region of liver.

---

* In regard to the pronunciation of words ending in *cele*, we may state, that
they may be treated as Latin words and the suffix pronounced *ce′le* or as English
words, in which case the suffix is pronounced *cel.*

hy'drocele, a protruding sac containing serum.
is'chiocele, hernia through inchiadic foramen.
menin'gocele, protrusion of meninges.
os'cheocele, scrotal hernia.
proc'tocele, hernia of rectum, prolapse of bowel.
sar'cocele, a fleshy enlargement of testicle.
splanch'nocele, a protrusion of any abdominal viscus.
trache'ocele, lit. a hernia in region of trachea, *goitre*.

8. -ec'tomy. Greek ἐκτομία, from ἐκτέμνω, to cut
out, a *cutting, extirpation.* This suffix is employed to
form words signifying the total removal of the part or
organ specified by the primitive. It differs from the
suffix -*tomy*, weich denotes the operation of *cutting*, but
not necessarily of cutting out or removal. The Latin
equivalent of ἐκτομία is *exsectio*.

arthrectomy, exsection of a joint.
chondrectomy, resection of a cartilage.
cionectomy, ablation of uvula.
coccygectomy, exsection of coccyx.
clitorectomy, ablation of clitoris.
corectomy, cutting out a part of the iris.
glossectomy, extirpation of the tongue.
hysterectomy, extirpation of uterus.
laryngectomy, extirpation of larynx.
nephrectomy, extirpation of kidney.
neurectomy, exsection of a portion of a nerve.
oophorectomy, extirpation of ovary.
orchiectomy, extirpation of testicle, castration.
ophthalmectomy, removal of eyeball.
phacectomy, removal of crystalline lens.
proctectomy, removal of portion of rectum.
pylorectomy, resection of pylorus.
splenectomy, removal of spleen.

9. **-graphy.** Greek γραφία, from γράφω, to write. A suffix denoting *description* of the thing designated by the primitive. *-graph* denotes an instrument for recording the movements of an organ; *-grapher*, one who writes about or describes a thing.

car′diograph, an instrument for recording the movements of the heart.

my′ograph, an instrument for recording movements of muscles.

sphyg′mograph, an instrument for recording the vibrations of an artery, fr. σφυγμός, pulse.

adenog′raphy, a description of the glands.

climatog′raphy, a description of climates (κλίμα).

cytog′raphy, a description of cells (κύτος).

desmog′raphy, a description of ligaments.

demog′raphy, a description of a people, vital statistics.

embryog′raphy, a description of embryos.

ethnog′raphy, a description of races or nations.

hæmatog′raphy, a description of the blood.

myog′raphy, a description of muscles, recording muscular movements.

neurog′raphy, a description of nervous diseases.

nosog′raphy, a description of diseases.

pharmacog′raphy, a description of drugs.

sphyg′mography, the art of using the sphygmograph.

syphilog′raphy, a description of syphititic lesions.

10. **-ia.** (Greek ια.) The Greek medical writers added this termination to the stem of a word designating an organ to denote a morbid condition of that organ. This termination is not much employed at present in the formation of new words, but a number of words thus formed have come down to us with meanings more or less changed.

ade'nia, disease of the lymphatic glands.

hyste'ria, originally womb disease, now a nervous affection.

me'tria, originally womb disease, now puerperal fever.

ophthal'mia, originally eye disease, now inflammation of the eye.

onych'ia, originally nail disease, now felon or whitlow.

pneumo'nia, originally lung disease, now inflammation of lungs.

diphthe'ria, originally disease of the membranes (διφθέρα) now an infectious disease with formation of false membrane.

11. -ic. Greek -ικός. A suffix used in the formation of adjectives, and denoting *pertaining* or *belonging to* the thing specified by the primitive. It is equivalent to the Latin -*alis* and -*icus*. The following are a few adjectives thus formed: —

caustic, burning, from καίω, to burn.

chronic, enduring, from χρόνος, time.

clonic, belonging to irregular spasm, fr. κλόνος, tumult.

eclec'tic, selective, from ἐκλέγω, to select.

enthet'ic, inoculable, from ἐντίθημι, to put in.

esoter'ic, pertaining to the organism, fr. ἐσώτερος, within.

hero'ic, belonging to a hero (ἥρως), applied to extreme methods of treatment.

idiopath'ic, belonging to a disease (πάθος) originating within one's self (ἴδιος), not acquired from without.

mephit'ic, belonging to a skunk (μεφίς), stinking.

picric, bitter (πικρός).

pol'iclinic, a city (πόλις) clinic.

polyclin'ic, a clinic with many beds or departments.

sporad ic, lit. sown, from σπείρω, to sow; not epidemic.

sthenic, pertaining to strength (σθένος), strong.
styptic, astringent, from στύφω, to contract.
tonic, making tense, firm, strong, from τείνω, to stretch.
trophic, nourishing, from τρέφω, to nourish.

12. -i'tis.   Greek -ῖτις.   This suffix was originally
a simple adjective termination like *-ic*, and was used with
νόσος, disease.   For example, νεφρής, feminine νεφρῖτις,
means belonging to the kidneys, and we find the word
so used by Hippocrates and Thucydides.   'Η γαστρῖτις
νόσος meant "the stomach complaint," ἡ νεφρῖτις νόσος
" the kidney complaint."   At a later period the word
νόσος, disease, was usually omitted.   During the present
century, and especially in all recent nosologies, this
suffix is employed to designate an inflammation of the
part specified by the primitive word.

adeni'tis, inflammation of a gland.
antri'tis, inflammation of antrum of Highmore.
aorti'tis, inflammation of aorta.
arteri'tis, inflammation of an artery.
arthri'tis, inflammation of a joint.
balani'tis, inflammation of glans penis.
blephari'tis, inflammation of eyelids.
bronchi'tis, inflammation of bronchi.
cardi'tis, inflammation of heart.
chondri tis, inflammation of a cartilage.
cioni tis, inflammation of uvula.
clitori tis, inflammation of clitoris.
coli'tis, inflammation of colon.
colpi'tis, inflammation of vagina.
cysti tis, inflammation of bladder.
dactyli'tis, syphilitic enlargement of fingers (a word
          coined by Bumstead).
dermati'tis, inflammation of skin.

dacryocysti′tis, inflammation of lachrymal sac.
dacryosoleni′tis, inflammation of lachrymal duct.
elytri′tis, inflammation of vagina.
epididymi′tis, inflammation of epididymis.
encephali′tis, inflammation of brain substance.
enteri′tis, inflammation of intestine.
gastri′tis, inflammation of stomach.
glossi′tis, inflammation of tongue.
hepati′tis, inflammation of liver.
hymeni′tis, inflammation of hymen.
ini′tis, inflammation of muscular fibres.
isthmi′tis, inflammation of fauces.
kerati′tis, inflammation of cornea.
laryngi′tis, inflammation of larynx.
masti′tis, inflammation of breast.
meningi′tis, inflammation of meninges.
metopantri′tis, inflammation of frontal sinuses.
metri′tis, inflammation of womb.
myosi′tis, inflammation of muscles.
myeli′tis, inflammation of marrow or spinal cord.
nephri′tis, inflammation of kidney.
neuri′tis, inflammation of a nerve.
nymphi′tis, inflammation of labia minora.
œsophagi′tis, inflammation of œsophagus.
oophori′tis, inflammation of ovaries.
orchi′tis, inflammation of testicle.
ostei′tis, inflammation of bone.
ophthalmi′tis, inflammation of globe of eye.
oti′tis, inflammation of ear.
pachymeningi′tis, inflammation of dura mater.
paranephri′tis, inflammation of suprarenal capsule.
paroti′tis, inflammation of parotid glands, mumps.
pancreati′tis, inflammation of pancreas.
peritoni′tis, inflammation of peritonæum.

phalli′tis, inflammation of penis.
phaci′tis, inflammation of crystalline lens.
phacocysti′tis, inflammation of capsule of lens.
pharyngi′tis, inflammation of pharynx.
phlebi′tis, inflammation of a vein.
pleuri′tis, inflammation of the pleura.
pneumoni′tis, inflammation of lungs.
pylephlebi′tis, inflammation of portal vein.
procti′tis, inflammation of rectum.
poliomyeli′tis, gray (πόλιος) inflammation of spinal cord.
posthi′tis, inflammation of foreskin.
pyeli′tis, inflammation of pelvis of kidney.
rachi tis, inflammation of spine; rickets.
rhini′tis, inflammation of nose.
salpingi′tis, inflammation of tube (Fallopian or Eusta-
　　chian).
spleni′tis, inflammation of spleen.
spondyli′tis, inflammation of a vertebra.
staphyli tis, inflammation of uvula.
stomati′tis, inflammation of mouth.
syndesmi′tis, inflammation of a ligament.
trachei′tis, inflammation of trachea.
tracheli tis, inflammation of neck of womb.
typhli′tis, inflammation of cæcum.
uli′tis, inflammation of gums.
uranisci′tis, inflammation of palate.
ureteri′tis, inflammation of ureter.
urethri′tis, inflammation of urethra.

13. -logy. Greek λογία, from λόγος, a word, dis-
course, or treatise. This suffix is added to the stems of
words to form compounds denoting a scientific treatise
on, or the science of the thing designated by the
primitive.

adenol ogy, a treatise on glands.

ætiol ogy, a treatise on the causes of disease.

angeiol ogy, a treatise on vessels.

arteriol ogy, a treatise on arteries.

arthrol ogy, a treatise on joints.

bacteriol'ogy, a treatise on bacteria (βακτηρία).

biol'ogy, a treatise on life, or the science of life.

chondrol'ogy, a treatise on cartilages.

climatol'ogy, a treatise on climates.

craniol ogy, a treatise on the skull or skulls.

dendrol'ogy, a treatise on trees (δένδρον).

dermatol ogy, the science treating of the skin.

eccrinol ogy, the science treating of secretions (ἔκκρισις).

embryol ogy, the science treating of embryos.

encephalol ogy, the science treating of the brain.

epidemiol ogy, the science treating of epidemics.

ethnol'ogy, the science treating of races or nations (ἔθνος).

gastrol'ogy, the science treating of the stomach.

glossol'ogy, the science treating of the tongue or of
  words.

gynæcol'ogy, the science treating of diseases of women
  (γύνη, a woman).

hæmol'ogy, the science treating of the blood.

helminthol'ogy, the science treating of intestinal worms
  (ἕλμινς).

histol'ogy, the science treating of tissues (ἱστόν).

homol'ogy, a treatise on corresponding parts or organs.

hydrol'ogy, a treatise on water.

hymenol'ogy, a treatise on membranes.

hypnol ogy, a treatise on sleep.

iamatol ogy, the science treating of remedies materia
  medica.

laryngol'ogy, the science treating of the larynx or throat.

loimol ogy, the science treating of plagues (λοιμός).

mastol'ogy, the science treating of the breast.

microbiol'ogy, the science treating of minute organisms.

morphol'ogy, the science treating of forms ($\mu o\mu\varphi\acute{\eta}$).

myol ogy, the science treating of muscles.

myxol'ogy, the science treating of mucous membranes.

necrol'ogy, a science treating of the dead members of a society.

nephrol'ogy, a treatise on the kidneys.

neurol'ogy, the science treating of the nerves and their diseases.

nosol'ogy, the science treating of the classification of diseases.

odontol'ogy, the science treating of the teeth.

oncol'ogy, the science treating of tumors.

ophthalmol'ogy, the science treating of the eyes.

osteol ogy, the science treating of bones.

otol'ogy, the science treating of the ears.

pædol'ogy, the science treating of children and their diseases.

parasitol'ogy, the science treating of parasites.

pathol'ogy, the science treating of diseases ($\pi\acute{a}\vartheta o\varsigma$).

phallol'ogy, the science treating of the penis.

pharmacol'ogy, the science treating of the action of drugs.

phonol'ogy, the science treating of the voice.

physiol'ogy, the science treating of growth, or life, ($\varphi\acute{v}\sigma\iota\varsigma$).

phytol'ogy, the science treating of plants, ($\varphi\upsilon\tau\acute{o}\nu$).

posol'ogy, the science treating of dose, fr. $\pi\upsilon\sigma\acute{o}\varsigma$, how much?

proctol ogy, the science treating of the rectum and anus.

psychol'ogy, the science treating of the mind, ($\psi\upsilon\chi\acute{\eta}$).

rhinol'ogy, the science treating of the nose.

spermatol'ogy, the science treating of the semen.

splanchnol'ogy, the science treating of the viscera.

semeiol'ogy, the science treating of signs and symptoms, fr. $\sigma\acute{\eta}\mu\varepsilon\iota o\nu$, a sign.

symptomatol'ogy, the science treating of symptoms of disease.

syndesmol'ogy, a treatise on ligaments.

tenontol'ogy, a treatise on tendons.

teratol'ogy, a treatise on monstrosities, (τέρας, a monster).

toxicol'ogy, a treatise on poisons, (τόξικον).

traumatol'ogy, a treatise on wounds.

urol'ogy, a treatise on the urine.

zymol'ogy, a treatise on ferments.

14. **-malacia.** Greek μαλαχία, softness, from μαλαχός, soft. This word, equivalent to the Latin *mollities*, is employed as a suffix to denote an abnormal softening of the part designated by the primitive.

cardiomala'cia, softening of tissues of the heart.

chondromala'cia, softening of a cartilage.

gastromala'cia, softening of walls of stomach.

hysteromalac'ia, or **hysteromalaco'ma,** softening of tissue of womb.

keratomala'cia, softening of the cornea.

myelomala'cia, softening of spinal cord.

osteomala'cia, softening of bones, mollities ossium.

phacomala'cia, softening of the crystalline lens.

splenomala'cia, softening of the spleen.

15. **-ma'nia.** Greek μανία, madness, a word akin to μήν, the moon, which the ancients supposed to be the cause of insanity. Mania is commonly derived from μένος, mind, whence, μνάομαι, to remember. It is used as a suffix in which the primitive has an adjective signification, denoting a prominent symptom of the mania.*

---

* We occasionally meet with such words as *morphinomania* and *cacainomania* denoting a morbid condition of the nervous system caused by morphine or cocaine. These words should not be admitted to our vocabularies, for aside from being hybrids, they are used to designate diseases in which there are no well-marked delusions. This latter objection applies also to *methomania* and *œnomania* when applied to cases in which drunkenness is the cause and not the result of the mental aberration.

dæmonoma'nia, insanity in which the patient believes himself to be possessed of devils (δαιμών).

dipsoma nia, insanity with excessive thirst (δίψα) for alcohol.

erotoma nia, a mania for loving the opposite sex; from Ἔρως, Cupid.

hysteroma'nia, hysterical mania.

kleptoma'nia, mania in which theft is the prominent symptom, from κλέπτω, to steal.

methoma'nia, insanity in which the patient has an uncontrollable desire to become intoxicated; fr. μεθύ, drunkenness.

nymphoma'nia, mania of women for sexual intercourse.

œnoma nia, same as *methomania,* fr. οἶνος, wine.

pyroma nia, insanity in which the patient sets buildings on fire, from πῦρ, fire.

theoma nia, religious insanity, from θεός, god.

16. **-odyn'ia.** Greek ὀδυνία, from ὀδύνη, severe physical pain, like Latin *dolor* and Sanskrit *du.* It is used as a suffix and attached to the stem of the word designating the location of the pain.

arthrodyn'ia, pain in a joint.

cardiodyn'ia, pain in the heart.

coccyodyn'ia, pain in coccygeal region.

gastrodyn'ia, pain in stomach.

metrodyn'ia, pain in womb.

mastodyn'ia, pain in breast.

ophthalmodyn'ia, pain in eye.

phallodyn'ia, pain in penis.

pleurodyn'ia, pain in side or pleura.

17. **-œde'ma.** Greek οἴδημα, a swelling, from οἰδέω, to swell. This word is used as a suffix to denote a swelling due to the infiltration of lymph, unless other-

wise specified by the primitive. It is attached (1) to the
stems of words designating the fluid which causes the
swelling, and (2) to the stems of words designating the
part where the swelling exists. It is not considered to
be in good taste to use this suffix in the formation of the
latter class of compounds which are necessarily words
of many syllables. "*Œdema of the brain*," for example,
is preferable to *encephalœdema*.

(1) **hydrœdema**, infiltration of tissues with watery fluid.
   lymphœdema, infiltration of tissues with lymph.
   myxœdema, infiltration of tissues with a substance
       resembling mucus (μύξα).

(2) **blepharœdema**, infiltration of tissues of eyelids.
   nymphœdema, infiltration of tissues of labia minora.
   phallœdema, infiltration of tissues of penis.
   pneumonœdema, infiltration of tissues of lungs.

18. **-oid.** Greek -οιδής or -ωδής, from εἶδος, a form
or image. This is an adjective suffix Latinized into
-*odes*, -*oides*, or -*oidalis*, and is the exact equivalent of
Latin -*formis*, from *forma*, a shape, or the English
shaped, like.

ad′enoid, gland-like.
an′thropoid, man-like or man-shaped, fr. ἄνθρωπος, man.
cesto′des, girdle-like, fr. κεστός, a girdle.
chon′droid, cartilage-like.
cho′roid, leather-like.
cir′soid, like a varix (κιρσός).
cli′noid, bed-like, fr. κλίνη, a couch.
col′loid, glue-like, fr. κόλλα, glue.
con′choid, shell-shaped, fr. κογχή, a shell.
co′noid, cone-shaped, fr. κῶνος, a cone.
cor′acoid, crow-bill-shaped, fr. κόραξ, a raven or crow.
17

cor'onoid, crown-like, fr. κορώνη, a crown.

cot'yloid, cup-shaped, fr. κοτύλη, a cup.

cri'coid, ring-shaped, fr. κρίκος, a ring.

cu'boid, cube-shaped, fr. κύβος, a cube.

del'toid, delta-shaped, *i. e.* like Δ.

der'moid, skin-like.

des'moid, ligament-like.

enceph'aloid, like brain tissue.

eth'moid, sieve-like, fr. ἠθμός, a sieve.

gle'noid, cave-like, fr. γλήνη, a cavity.

hæm'atoid, blood-like.

ha'loid, salt-like, fr. ἅλς, salt, or the sea.

hel'coid, ulcer-like, fr. ἕλκος, an ulcer.

hy'aloid, glass-like, from ὕαλος, glass.

hy'oid, upsilon-shaped, like υ.

hys'teroid, hysteria-like.

ke'loid, tumor-like, resembling a rupture (κηλή).

lamb'doid, lambda-shaped, *i. e.* like Λ.

lep'idoid, scale-like, from λεπίς, a scale.

mas'toid, breast or nipple-shaped.

my'oid, muscle-like.

na'noid, dwarf-like, from νᾶνος, a dwarf.

nem'atoid, thread-like, from νῆμα, a thread.

neph'roid, kidney-shaped.

odon'toid, tooth-like.

os'teoid, bone-like.

pter'ygoid, wing-like, aliform, from πτέρυξ, a wing.

rheu'matoid, like rheumatism.

ses'amoid, like a sesame seed.

sig'moid, sigma-shaped, *i. e.* like ς.

sphe'noid, wedge-shaped, from σφήν, a wedge.

tet'anoid, like tetanus.

thy'roid, shield-shaped, from θυρεός, a shield.

trap'ezoid, table-like, from τράπεζα, a table.

ty'phoid, like typhus, from τῦφος, stupor.

xiph'oid, sword-like, from ξίφον, a sword.

19. -o'ma. Greek -ωμα. This is an inseparable suffix used in the formation of nouns from verbs (verbal nouns). It denotes the result of the action of the verb. Thus, from κάρκινος, a crab, Latin *cancer*, the verb καρκινόω, to have a cancer, is formed, and from this verb is derived καρκίνωμα (*carcinoma*) the result of the cancerous process, the cancerous tumor. Many of the verbs denoting morbid processes in Greek end in όω, and from these, verbal nouns designating the result of the action expressed by the verb, are formed by adding -ωμα, -oma, to the stem. In cases where this termination is apparently added to a noun stem, the intermediate formation of a verb is understood. For example, *adeno'ma* is not derived directly from ἀδήν, a gland, but from ἀδενόω, to form a gland, and *adenoma* means a gland-like formation or tumor. -o'ma is now limited to the construction of words designating tumors formed as the result of morbid processes and malignant growths of all kinds.

atheroma, a groat-like tumor, fr. ἀθήρα, groats.

angeioma, a vascular tumor, fr. ἀγγεῖον, a vessel.

cephaloma, a brain-like tumor, fr. κεφαλή, head.

cephalhæmatoma, a blood tumor on the head.

chondroma, a cartilaginous tumor.

dermatoma, a cutaneous tumor.

encephaloma, a brain-like tumor.

enchondroma, a cartilaginous tumor from bone.

epithelioma, an epithelial tumor.

glioma, a glue-like tumor, from γλία, glue.

hæmatoma, a tumor containing blood.

inoma, a fibrous tumor, from ἴς, fibre.

keratoma, a horny tumor, from κέρας, a horn.

leucoma, a white tumor, from λευκός, white.

lipoma, a fatty tumor.

melanoma, a black pigmentary tumor.

myoma, a muscular tumor.

myxoma, a tumor composed of mucous tissue.

neuroma, a nerve tumor.

odontoma, a dental tumor.

osteoma, a bony tumor.

othæmatoma, a blood tumor of ear, hæmatoma auris.

sarcoma, a malignant fleshy tumor.

scleroma, a hard tumor, from σκληρός, hard.

staphyloma, a grape-like tumor, i. e. projection of cornea.

steatoma, a tumor containing stiff fat.

sycoma, a fig-like excrescence, fr. σῦκον, a fig.

trachoma, rough (τραχύς) swelling of eyelid, or conjunctiva.

xanthoma, a yellow fibrous tumor, fr. ξανθός, yellow.

20. **on'cus.** Greek ὄγκος, a word meaning, primarily, a weight, from ἄγκω, to bend (the arm of a balance); cognate with Sanskrit *ankami*, with Latin *uncus*, a hook, and *uncia*, an ounce, and with English *ankle*, the bend between leg and foot. As a suffix -*on'cus* has the secondary meaning of a tumor or mass without regard to its origin, a non-malignant tumor; thus differing from -*oma* which designates a tumor resulting from a morbid process and -*cele* which denotes ordinarily a tumor due to the misplacement of a viscus. -*oncus* is added to the stem of the noun which designates the location of the tumor.

arthroncus, a tumor in a joint; floating cartilage.

episeioncus, a tumor in pubic region, or of labia, from ἐπίσειον, pubes.

hepatoncus, a tumor of the liver.

mastoncus, a tumor of the breast.

pancreatoncus, a tumor of the pancreas.
phalloncus, a tumor of the penis.
splenoncus, a tumor of the spleen.
uloncus, a tumor of the gums.

21. **-o'pia.** Greek -ωπία, from ὤψ, the eye or eye-sight, from ὄπτω, to see. *-opsia*, Greek -ωψία, from the same. These are used as suffixes to the stems of words used adjectively denoting the kind of sight or defect of vision.

amblyopia, defective or weak sight, fr. ἀμβλύς, blunted.
ametropia, abnormal (ἀμέτρον, out of measure) sight.
asthenopia, weak (ἀσθενής) sight.
copyopia, weary sight, from κόπος, weary.
diplopia, double (δίπλοον) sight, seeing double.
emmetropia, normal (ἐμμέτρον, in measure) vision.
hemeralopia, sight by day only, fr. ἡμέρα, day.
hæmatopsia, blood-colored vision.
hyperopia, over (ὑπέρ) vision; far sight.
myopia, fr. μύω, to shut the eyes; a symptom of near-sightedness; near sight.
micropsia, vision in which objects appear smaller than they are.
megalopsia, vision in which objects appear larger than they are.
xanthopsia, yellow vision, from ξανθός, yellow.

22. **-pathy.** Greek πάθια, from πάθος, an affection, disease. This suffix is used in two ways: (1) it is attached to the stems of nouns to denote a diseased condition of the part designated by primitive, and (2) to the stems of adjectives or words used adjectively to form compounds denoting a system of treatment.

(1) **adenop'athy,** diseased condition of lymphatic glands
     cardiop'athy, diseased condition of heart.
     hysterop'athy, diseased condition of womb.
     neurop'athy, a diseased condition of nervous system.
     psychop'athy, a diseased condition of mind.

(2) **allop'athy,** a word coined by Hahnemann to denote
         means of cure otherwise than by *homœo-*
         pathy, fr. *ἄλλος,* other.
     dæmonop'athy, cure by invoking the aid of spirits,
         fr. *δαιμών,* spirit.
     electrop'athy, cure by use of electricity.
     homœop'athy, cure by using remedies producing
         symptoms like (*ὅμοιος*) those of the disease.
     hydrop'athy, cure by using water.
     theop'athy, cure by invoking God(*θεός*); prayer cure.

23. **-pho bia.** Greek *-φοβία,* from *φόβος,* fear, or
φοβέω, to be afraid. This suffix is used to form words
denoting the symptom of morbid fear. It is attached to
the stem of the word which designates that of which
the patient is afraid.

agoraphobia, fear of the market place (*ἀγορά*); of being
     alone in large places.
anthropophobia, dread of society, man-kind (*ἄνθρωπος*).
cynophobia, morbid fear of dogs (*κύων*).
cypriphobia, fear of sexual intercourse, fr. *Κυπρίς,* Venus.
kenophobia, fear of empty places, fr. *κενός,* empty.
hydrophobia, fear of water, a misnomer for *rabies.*
mysophobia, fear of contamination, from *μυσός,* dirt.
photophobia, dread or intolerance of light.
pyrophobia, fear of fire.
syphiliphobia, morbid fear of contracting syphilis.

24. **·plas'ty.** Greek -πλαστία, from πλάσσω, to mould. This suffix denotes the operation by which the part designated by the primitive is restored. If the tissue is taken from the patient the operation is called *autoplasty*, if from another, *heteroplasty*, from ἕτερος, other.

blepharoplasty, restoration of eyelid.

cheiloplasty, restoration of lip.

cystoplasty, restoration of walls of bladder.

dermoplasty, restoration of skin; skin grafting.

elytroplasty, restoration of the vaginal walls.

gastroplasty, restoration of walls of stomach.

gnathoplasty, restoration of the tissues on jaw or cheek.

helcoplasty, restoration of skin over an ulcer (ἕλκος).

keratoplasty, restoration of cornea.

oscheoplasty, restoration of scrotal sac.

perinæoplasty, restoration of perinæum.

rhinoplasty, restoration of nose.

urethroplasty, restoration of urethra.

25. **-rhaphy.** Greek ῥαφία, from ῥαφή, a suture or seam, from ῥάπτω, to sew or stitch. Thus we speak of the *rhaphe perinæi* and *rhaphe occipitis*, because these parts appear to have been stitched together. The suffix *-rhaphy* denotes the operation of suturing the part designated by the primitive.

elytror'rhaphy, suturing the vagina.

enteror'rhaphy, suturing an intestine.

neuror'rhaphy, suturing a nerve.

perinæor'rhaphy, suturing the perinæum.

proctor'rhaphy, suturing the rectum or anus.

staphylor'rhaphy, lit. suturing the uvula (σταφυλή); a mis-
        nomer for suturing the palate for cleft palate.

trachelor'rhaphy, suturing the neck of uterus.

uraniscor'rhaphy, suturing the palate for cleft palate.

26. **-rha'gia.** Greek ῥαγία, from ῥήγνυμι, to burst forth. This suffix is attached to stems of words, (1) to denote an excessive flow of blood from the part designated by the primitive, or (2) to denote an excessive flow of the substance designated by the primitive. In the former class it may usually be translated *hemorrhage of.*

blennorrhagia, an excessive discharge of mucus; gonorrhœa.

clitorrhagia, hemorrhage from clitoris.

enterrhagia, hemorrhage from bowels.

hæmorrhagia, an abnormal flow of blood.

menorrhagia, an excessive flow of menstrual blood.

metrorrhagia, hemorrhage from the womb, not menstrual.

nymphorrhagia, a hemorrhage from the labia minora.

phallorrhagia, a hemorrhage from the penis.

pharyngorrhagia, a hemorrhage from the pharynx.

rhinorrhagia, a hemorrhage from the nose.

ulorrhagia, a hemorrhage from the gums.

27. **-rhœ'a.** Greek ῥοία, from ῥέω, to flow, equivalent to the Latin *fluxus,* from *fluo,* to flow. This suffix, when attached to the stems of nouns designating parts of the body, denotes an abnormal flow of mucus (catarrh) or other secretion from the part specified by the primitive. It is also attached to the stems of words used adjectively describing the nature of the flux.

blennorrhœa, an abnormal discharge of mucus.

bronchorrhœa, catarrh of the bronchi.

catarrh, a flowing down (κατά); excessive discharge of mucus.

cystorrhœa, catarrh of the bladder.

colporrhœa, vaginal catarrh.

diarrhœa, flowing through (διά) of contents of intestines.

emmenorrhœa, monthly flow, menses.

enterorrhœa, catarrh of intestines.

galactorrhœa, excessive flow of milk.

gastrorrhœa, catarrh of stomach.

gonorrhœa, flow of semen; misnomer for blennorrhagia.

hydrorrhœa, watery discharge.

laryngorrhœa, catarrh of larynx.

leucorrhœa, white (λευκός) discharge from vagina.

metrorrhœa, catarrh of uterus.

ophthalmorrhœa, catarrh of eyes.

orrhorrhœa, discharge of serum (ὄῤῥος).

otorrhœa, catarrh of ear.

phallorrhœa, mucous discharge from penis.

pharyngorrhœa, catarrh of pharynx.

piarrhœa, excessive flow from sebaceous glands.

proctorrhœa, catarrh of rectum.

rhinorrhœa, nasal catarrh.

salpingorrhœa, catarrh of Eustachian tube.

spermatorrhœa, abnormal flow of semen.

trachelorrhœa, catarrh of cervix uteri.

28. **-sis.** Greek σις. A suffix used in forming verbal nouns. It is equivalent to the Latin *-ens*, *-entia*, *-cia*, and English *-ing*, and denotes a process, action, or possession. It is added to the stems of verbs to form nouns denoting the continuance of such action, process, or possession. Thus from ἄνθραξ, coal, we have the verb ἀνθρακόω, to turn to coal, and ἀνθράκωσις, a turning to coal, now applied to the deposit of coal dust in the lungs, or to the formation of carbuncles (ἄνθρακες) which were supposed to resemble coals. So also *carcinosis* denotes the cancerous process, formation of cancer, as *carcinoma* denotes the result of the process, a cancerous tumor.

amauro sis, a darkening, blindness, fr. ἀμαυρόω, to darken

archebio sis, original (ἀρχή, beginning) formation of life, from βιω, to live.

argyro'sis, lit. a turning silver; a deposit of silver salts in tissues.

biogen'esis, generation of life, fr. βιογεννάω, to form life.

byssino sis, lit. a turning to cotton (βύσσος); deposit of cotton in lungs.

cardiec tasis, dilatation of heart, fr. ἐκτάω, to distend.

chemo sis, lit. formation of a cavity (χήμη); inflammation of eyes in which the cornea seems to be in a cavity.

chloro'sis, a turning greenish yellow, from χλωρόω, to turn green.

chromidro sis, having colored sweat, fr. χρωμός, colored.

cirrho sis, turning reddish yellow, from κιρρόω, to turn reddish yellow.

copho'sis, deafness, from κοφόω, to be deaf.

coreclei sis, closing of the pupil, from κορηκλείω, to close

cyano'sis, turning blue (κύανος).

cyrto sis, a bending, from κυρτόω, to bend.

dermatol'ysis, a shedding of the skin, from δερματολύω, to cast off the skin.

distichi'asis, having a double row (διστιχος) of eyelashes.

dosis, dose, a giving, fr. δίδωμι, to give.

ecchymo'sis, a pouring out of blood into the tissues, fr. ἐγχυμόω, to pour out.

elephanti asis, becoming like an elephant (ἐλεφαντιάζω); a disease in which there is great hypertrophy of tissues.

gompho sis, (articulating) like a molar tooth, fr. γομφόω, to cut teeth.

hæmatem'esis, a vomiting of blood, fr. αἱματεμέω.

helco sis, ulceration, fr. ἑλκόω, to ulcerate.

helminthi asis, having intestinal worms, from ἑλμινθιάζω, to have worms.

histol ysis, dissolution of tissue.

hystrici'asis, resembling a hedgehog (ὕστριξ); stiffness of the hair.

icthyo'sis, resembling a fish (ἰχθύς); scaly skin disease.

iridokine'sis, abnormal movement or twitching of iris.

lithi'asis, formation of calculi (λίθοι).

lordo'sis, a bending forward of spine, from λορδόω, to bow down.

lysis, solution, breaking up of a disease, fr. λύω, to loose.

narco'sis, stupefaction, from ναρκόω, to stupefy.

necro'sis, a dying, mortification, fr. νεκρόω, to mortify.

pathogen'esis, generation of a disease.

phimo'sis, a muzzling (of penis with foreskin) fr. φιμόω, to muzzle.

phlegmo'sis or **-ma'sia,** inflammation, from φλεγμάζω, to inflame.

phtheiri'asis, having lice, fr. φθειριάζω, to have lice.

phthisis, a wasting, fr. φθίω, to waste away.

pityri'asis, scurfiness, fr. πιτυριάζω, to be scurfy.

polio'sis, turning gray of hair, fr. πολιόω, to become gray.

poro'sis, a hardening, callous, fr. πωρόω, to harden.

psori'asis, having the itch, fr. ψωρά; a squamous skin disease.

ptosis, a falling, drooping of the eyelid, fr. πίπτω, to fall.

pyro'sis, a burning (in the stomach), fr. πυρόω, to set on fire.

rhachiocamp'sis, spinal curvature, fr. κάμπτω, to curve.

rhachiocypho'sis, having a hump back, fr. κυφόω, to make a hump.

rhexis, a rupture of a vessel, fr. ῥήγνυμι, to burst.

rhutido'sis, a wrinkling (of cornea before death), fr. ῥυτιδόω, to wrinkle.

satyri'asis, acting like a satyr, inordinate sexual desire, fr. σατυριάζω, to play the satyr.

scolio'sis, curvature (of spine), fr. σκολιόω, to be crooked.

trichi'asis, having hairs, eyelashes growing into eyes, fr. θρίξ, a hair.

trichino'sis, being affected with trichinæ.

zymo'sis, fermentation, an infectious process, fr. ζυμόω, to make yeast, to ferment.

29. **-scopy.** Greek -σκοπία, from σκοπέω, to examine. A word derived from σκέπτομαι, to look at, like Latin *inspectio*, from *specio*. This suffix denotes the act of examining the part specified by the primitive. It is equivalent to the Latin *spectio.*

elytros'copy, the examination of the vagina.

endos'copy, the examination of cavities, parts within.

gastros'copy, the examination of the stomach.

gynæcos'copy, the examination of female genitals.

laryngos'copy, the examination of the larynx.

micros'copy, the examination of small things.

ophthalmos'copy, the examination of the eye.

otos'copy, the examination of the ear.

pharyngos'copy, the examination of the throat.

proctos'copy, the examination of the rectum.

rhinos'copy, the examination of the nose.

stethos'copy, the examination of the chest.

urethros'copy, the examination of the urethra.

All of the words ending in *-scopy* signify an ocular examination, except *stethoscopy,* which denotes an examination by means of the ear.

30. **-s'mus.** Greek -σμος, English *-sm.* A termination added to the stems of intensive and frequentative verbs, *i. e.* those ending in ζω, to form verbal nouns. Thus, from σπάω, to draw, we form the intensive verb σπάζω, to draw hard, or with a frequentative sense, to draw often. From this verb we get σπάσμος, Latin *spas-*

mus, English *spasm.* As a termination it denotes that the action expressed by the verb takes place frequently or rapidly. A secondary meaning is irritability or spasm. With this signification it is attached to the stem of the noun designating the part affected. In a few cases, as in *aneurysm,* from ἀνευρύζω, to widen out, it has the same signification as the termination -*sis.*

erethism, irritability, from ἐριθίζω, to irritate.

rheumatism, lit. abounding in humors (ῥεύματα).

laryngismus, spasm of larynx, from λαρυγγίζω, to shout.

marasmus, a rapid wasting, fr. μαράζω, to waste away.

œsophagismus, spasm of œsophagus.

pharyngismus, spasm of pharynx.

priapism, constant or frequent erection of penis.

ptyalism, spitting frequently, salivation, fr. πτύω, to spit.

strabismus, squinting, fr. στραβίζω, to squint.

trachelismus, a throttling spasm of neck, fr. τραχηλίζω, to throttle.

tenesmus, a constant or severe straining (τενέζω, to strain severely).

trismus, a gnashing the teeth, lock-jaw, from τρίζω, to grate the teeth.

31. **-tomy.** Greek τομία, from τέμνω, to cut. A suffix equivalent to Latin *sectio,* cutting, used to form words denoting the operation of cutting the part designated by the primitive. As it means simply *incision,* it should not be applied to operations of cutting out, or removing a part. *Lithotomy,* for example, is a misnomer, for the stone is not *cut* but *cut out,* the bladder being the part incised. *Lithectomy* or *litho-cystotomy,* bladder cutting for stone, would have been better words to designate the operation.

amygdalot'omy, cutting the tonsils.
anat'omy, cutting up (ἀνά), dissection.
anthropot'omy, human anatomy.
arteriot'omy, section of an artery.
bronchot'omy, section of a bronchus.
chondrot'omy, cutting a cartilage.
cholecystot'omy, cutting the gall bladder.
cionot'omy, cutting the uvula.
colot'omy, cutting the colon.
craniot'omy, cutting the skull.
cystot'omy, cutting the bladder.
elytrot'omy, cutting the vagina.
embryot'omy, cutting the embryo or fœtal head.
enterot'omy, cutting the intestine.
hysterot'omy, cutting the womb.
keratot'omy, cutting the cornea.
laryngot'omy, cutting the larynx.
laparot'omy, cutting the loin.
laparo-elytrot'omy, cutting the loin and vagina.
myot'omy, cutting a muscle.
nephrot'omy, cutting into the kidney.
neurot'omy, cutting a nerve.
œsophagot'omy, cutting the œsophagus.
orchiot'omy, cutting a testicle.
osteot'omy, cutting a bone.
phacocystot'omy, cutting into the capsule of lens.
pharyngot'omy, cutting into the pharynx.
phlebot'omy, cutting into a vein, venesection.
pleurot'omy, cutting into the pleura or side.
pneumonot'omy, cutting into the lung.
proctot'omy, cutting into the rectum or anus.
rhachiot'omy, cutting the spine.
salpingot'omy, cutting the Fallopian tube.
staphylot'omy, cutting the uvula.

syndesmot'omy, cutting a ligament.
syringot'omy, cutting a fistula (σύριγξ).
tenot'omy, cutting a tendon.
tracheot'omy, cutting the trachea.
trachelot'omy, cutting neck of womb.
typhlot'omy, cutting the cæcum.
urethrot'omy, cutting the urethra.

32. **-u'ria.** English *-ury*, Greek *-ουρία*, from *ουρέω*, to urinate. This suffix is attached to the stems of words used adjectively to form compounds designating the various abnormalities of the urine and micturition.

anuria, total suppression of urine.
azoturia, excess of urea in urine, fr. *azote*, a name for nitrogen.
choluria, bile in the urine.
chyluria, chyle in the urine.
dysuria, difficult or painful urination.
galacturia, milk in the urine, or milk-white urine.
galactosuria, milk sugar in the urine.
glycosuria, glucose in the urine.
hæmaturia, blood in the urine.
hæmaglobinuria, hæmoglobin in the urine.
ischuria, suppression of urine, fr. *ἔχω*, to hold.
melanuria, black or dark colored urine.
mellituria, honey (*μελι*) in the urine, same as glycosuria.
oliguria, scanty urine.
polyuria, excessive excretions of urine.
pyuria, pus in the urine.
stran'gury, difficult urination, fr. *στράγξ*, a drop.

CHAPTER VI

ETYMOLOGY OF SOME OTHER WORDS OF GREEK ORIGIN.

acro'mion, fr. ἄκρον, top, and ὦμος, shoulder.

actinomyco'sis, from ἀκτίν, a ray, and μύκης, a fungus; radiating fungus.

æg'ilops, from αἴξ, a goat, and ὤψ, eye; ulcer in corner of eye.

ægoph'oy, fr. αἴξ, a goat, φωνή, voice; bleating sound.

allot'ropy, from ἄλλος, other, and τρέπω, to turn; changing to another form.

amal'gam, fr. ἅμα, together, γαμέω, to marry; mixture of metals.

alope'cia, from ἀλώπηξ, the fox, which is sometimes bald; baldness.

ankylo'sis, immobility, fr. ἀγκυλόω, to clasp.

ankylo-glos'sia, clasp (ἀγκυλή) tongue (γλῶσσα); tongue-tie.

anthropoph'agous, man eating, fr. ἄνθρωπος, man, and φάγω, to eat.

aphtha, fr. ἅπτω, to burn; a burning, sore mouth.

arach'noid, spider web-like membrane, from ἀράχνη, a spider.

asci'tes, a full bag (ἀσκίτης); abdominal dropsy.

asthma, a gasping for breath, from ἀσθμάζω, to gasp for breath.

atro'pa, fr. Ἄτροπος, the Fate that ends life; belladonna.

bacte'rium, fr. βακτήριον, a little rod; microbe.

bary'ta, heavy metal, fr. βαρύς, heavy.

basil'ikon, the royal (βασιλικός) ointment.

bi'oplasm, life-forming substance, fr. βίος, life, and πλάσσω, to form.

bot'any. fr. βοτάνη, an herb; the science of plants.
bothrioceph'alus, a tapeworm with the little pitted (βοθρίον) head.
bromine, the element with the bad smell, from βρῶμος, noisome.
bronchoph'ony, bronchial voice, fr. βρόγχος and φωνή.
brygmus, gnashing of teeth, fr. βρύζω, to gnash.
bulim'ia, fr. βοῦς, an ox; ravenous appetite.
ca'lyx, fr. κάλυξ, a cup.
ceph'alotribe, a head crusher, fr. κεφαλή, head, and τρείβω, to rub to powder.
chi'asm, formation of letter *chi* (X).
chloas'ma, formation of yellow color on skin, fr. χλωρός, yellow.
choled'ochus, gall receiver, fr. χολή, bile, and δέχομαι, to receive.
chol'era, lit. the bilious disease, ἡ χολερή (νόσος).
chore'a, fr. χοραία, a choral dance; St. Vitus' Dance.
chro'mium, fr. χρῶμα, color; the colored element.
clys'ter, that which washes away (κλυστήρ); enema.
coc'cus, fr. κόκκος, a berry; cochineal.
codei'na, fr. κωδεία, a poppy head; an alkaloid of opium.
col'lagen, the glue (κόλλα) making substance.
coma, fr. κόμη, a mask; stupor.
cory'za, fr. κόρση, forehead, and ζέω, to boil; cold in head.
cre'osote, κρέας, meat, and σώζω, to preserve; oil of smoke.
cre'atin, an extractive from flesh (κρέας).
cryptor'chis, having a concealed (κρυπτός) testicle (ὀρχίς).
dolichoceph'alus, having long (δολιχός) head (κεφαλή).
dynamom'eter, a force (δύναμις) measurer (μέτρον).
echinococ'cus, lit. a hedge-hog berry, fr. ἐχῖνος, a hedge-hog; embryo of tape worm.
emprosthot'onos, a stretching forward (ἔμπροσθεν) spasm.
en'terolith, stone-like fæces in intestine, fr. λίθος, a stone.
18

erythe'ma, redness of skin, fr. ἐρυθέω, to blush.

eschar, a scab from a burn, fr. ἐσχαρόω, to scab over.

eu'nuch, lit. a bed keeper, fr. εὐνή, a bed, and ἔχω, to keep.

gan'grene, lit. an eating away (γάγγραινα).

graph'ite, writing stone, plumbago, fr. γράφω, to write.

hæmop'tysis, spitting blood, fr. πτύω, to spit, and αἷμα, blood.

hem'orrhoid, resembling a flow of blood, first applied to bleeding piles, fr. αἱμαρῥέω, to flow blood.

hal'ogen, salt making, fr. ἅλς, salt, and γεννάω, to make.

hectic, habitual, constitutional, fr. ἕξις, a habit.

her'nia, dim. cf. ἔρνος, a breach, a rupture.

herpes, fr. ἕρπω, to creep; a skin disease, "shingles."

Hippoc'rates, lit. a horse driver, fr. ἵππος, a horse, and κρατέω, to govern, "the Father of Medicine.

hip'pus, a constant winking, as seen in the horse (ἵππος).

hy'datid, lit. a watery vesicle, fr. ὑδατίς, a cyst containing water.

hydroceph'alus, lit. water head (ὕδωρ and κεφαλή), dropsy of brain.

hy'drogen, water (ὕδωρ) making (γεννάω).

hydronephro'sis, watery collection about kidney.

hydropericar'dium, watery serum in pericardium.

hy'giene, fr. ὑγεία, health; cognate with Sanskrit *ugras*, strength. Hygeia was the daughter of Æsculapius.

hyphom'yces, web fungus, from ὕφος, a web, and μύκης, fungus.

idiosyn'crasy, from ἴδιος, one's own, συγκρᾶσις, mixing together; temperament.

i'odine, fr. ἰωδής, violet-like, fr. ἴον, a violet; an element.

kinesither'apy, movement (κίνησις) cure (θεραπεῖα).

kyes'tein or **cyes'tein,** from κύησις, pregnancy, and ἐσθής, clothing; a substance in urine of pregnant women.

lagophthal'mia, hare (λαγώς) eye; inability to close eye.

lagos'toma, hare (λαγώς) mouth (στόμα); harelip.

lec'ethin, a substance found in yolk of egg (λέκιθος) and brain.

lepra, lit. the scaly disease, fr. λέπος, a scale; leprosy.

lep'tothrix, lit. a delicate (λεπτός) hair (θρίξ); a microphyte.

leu'cocyte, a white cell or blood corpuscle from λευκός, white, κύτος, cell.

lupus, fr. λυπή, pain, contracted from *lypesis*, certainly not the Latin *lupus*, a wolf; painful eating ulcer.

lyssa, rabies, fr. λύσσα, madness.

macroscop'ic, seen from a distance, fr. μακρός, long.

melæ'na, black (μέλας) vomit.

melano'sis, deposit of black pigment; black jaundice.

melas'ma, blackness from a contusion.

mias'ma, a pollution of the air, fr. μιάζω, to pollute.

micrococ'cus, a small (μικρός) berry (κόκκος), spherobacterium.

neurilem'ma, nerve sheath or bark (λέμμα).

neurog'lia, nerve glue (γλία).

niphlotyphlo'tes, snow (νίφα) blindness (τυφλότης).

olec'ranon, (ὠλένη) ulna (κράνος) head.

orthoped'ic, fr. ὀρθόω, to straighten, and παῖς, a child.

orthopnœ'a, ὀρθός, upright position, and πνοία, breathing.

os'teoblast, a bone (ὀστέον) bud (βλάστημα).

o'tolith, a stone (λίθος) found in ear (οὖς).

oxyu'res, worms with sharp (ὀξύς) tails (οὐρα).

ozæ'na, the name of a stinking sea fish (ὀζαίνα); fetid nasal catarrh.

o'zone, fr. ὄζω, to stink; modified oxygen.

pachybleph'aron, thick (παχύς) eyelids (βλέφαρα).

pæd'erasty, unnatural love (ἐραστία) of boys (παῖδες).

pæd'iatry, the art of child (παῖς) curing (ἰατρεία).

pathet'ic, pertaining to the feelings (πάθοι).

pathognomon'ic, belonging to a symptom by which we know (γιγνώσκω) a disease.

pem'phigus, a skin disease characterized by blisters (πέμφιγες).

phagedæ'na, an eating sore, fr. φάγω, to eat.

phar'macy, the art of preparing drugs (φάρμακα).

pharmacopœ'a, lit. drug making, fr. ποιέω, to make.

phlyctæ'na, a blistered sore (φλύκταινα).

placen'ta, Latinized fr. πλακοῦς, a cake; afterbirth.

pleomas'tia, supernumerary nipples, fr. πλέος, more, and μαστός, breast.

pleth'ora, fullness, fr. πλῆθος, full.

pleurosthot'onos, a spasm (τόνος) drawing to the side (πλεύροσθεν).

ple'ximeter, a stroke (πλῆξις) measure (μέτρον).

pneumo-tho'rax, air (πνεῦμα) in the chest (θώραξ).

pom'pholyx, a bubble-like eruption on skin (πομφός, a bubble).

pseudoplas'ma, from ψευδής, false, abnormal (πλάσμα) formation.

pteryg'ium, a wing-like (πτέρυξ) growth on eyeball.

pto'maine, an alkaloid obtained from a corpse (πτῶμα).

pyotho'rax, pus (πύον) in the chest (θώραξ), *i. c.* in pleural cavity.

rhin'othrix, a nose hair (ῥίς, nose, θρίξ, hair).

rhoncus, a snoring sound (ῥόγχος).

sap'rophyte, a putrefactive (σαπρός) plant (φυτόν).

schizomyce'tes, splitting (σχίζω) fungi (μυκήτες).

scirrus, a hard (σκιρρός) tumor; stone cancer.

scolex, an embryo of tapeworm, fr. σκώληξ, a worm.

scyb'alum, a fœcal mass (σκύβαλον), fr. ἐς κύνας βάλλειν, to throw to the dogs; the scavengers of ancient cities.

sial'olith, salivary (σίαλον) calculus (λίθος).

skel'eton, fr. σκελετός, dried; framework.

tet'anus, lock-jaw, fr. τείνω, to stretch.

theca, a receptacle, sheath (θήκη).

thenar, palm, or sole (θέναρ), fr. θείνω, to strike.

therapeu'tics, from θεραπεύω, to wait upon, attend, cure; the science of curing diseases.

thrombus, a venous clot, fr. θρόμβος, a clot of blood.

tragus, a part of external ear covered with hair, from τράγος, a goat.

trichoceph'alus, a hair-headed parasite, from θρίξ, a hair, and κεφαλή, head.

trochan'ter, a roller, fr. τροχάω, to roll.

typhus, a fever with stupor (τῦφος).

tyrotox'icon, cheese (τυρός) poison (τοξικόν).

ulat'rophy, atrophy of gums (οὖλα, gum, ἀτροφία).

zoster, a girdle, zone, fr. ζωστήρ.

CHAPTER VII.

HYBRID WORDS.

HYBRID words are those derived from two languages, a method of formation regarded as unscientific by philologists. The word *hybrid* is derived from the Greek ὕβρις, wantonness, violence, or rape, through the Latin *hybrida* or *hibrida*, a mongrel, or a person born of a Roman father and foreign mother. The classical writers were exceedingly careful to avoid words formed in this manner, and the Grecian orator, although allowed to coin new words from his own tongue with the greatest liberty, would have been greeted with hisses if not a shower of stones, had he committed the dreadful crime of using a hybrid word, such as medical men use daily when talking of *albuminuria* or *asafœtida*. The Greeks called all foreigners barbarians, (βάρβαροι) not because they had long beards, *barbœ*, and needed the services of a barber, as is sometimes supposed, but because the languages of these strangers sounded to the Hellenic ear like *bah-bah-bah*, a kind of speech far beneath them. Demosthenes would no more have thought of forming a new word by uniting Greek and Latin than a Southern gentleman would think of marrying his daughter to the blackest negro on his plantation.

While the older classical medical terms were formed according to the strictest rules of etymology, many of these hybrids have of late been introduced into the language of medicine and taken a firm root in our literature. American physicians, particularly the specialists, are responsible for the great majority of these mongrels, possibly because of the cosmopolitan character of our nation, but more probably on account of the total lack of philological training in this country. The specialist derives nearly as much pleasure from the coining of a new word as from the invention of a new instrument, although he usually evinces far less skill in his etymological than in his mechanical inventions.

The language of a science should be scientific in all particulars, and all hybrid words should be relegated to "ϕυχοcurists," "ϖiταπαθιστες," and other nondescript practitioners. *Vaginitis*, for example, is quite as improperly formed as *digititis*, or *fingeritis*, yet *vaginitis* is used by the best medical scholars, while *fingeritis* or *nositis* would be ridiculed by the most illiterate of practitioners. With the dictionaries of Greece, Rome and France open for our use in selecting and forming new scientific words, there is no occasion for the introduction of these hybrids.

In a few instances it would be somewhat difficult to find a proper substitute for these hybrid words. *Albuminuria*, for example, is both euphonic and expressive, although composed of the Latin *albumen* and the Greek *-ουρια*. If we attempt to convert this into a pure Greek word we may have *synoruria*, from συνώFου, white of egg, or on the other hand, we might use the pure Latin, *albuminurina*.

We give below a list of common hybrids with their derivation and pure Greek equivalents, using quotation marks when the word is not found in the medical dictionaries.

antifeb'rine, fr. Gk. αντί, against, and Lat. *febris*, fever, antipyrine.*

cæci'tis, Lat. *cæcum* and Gk. ῖτις, typhlitis.

* As "antipyrine" is applied to a different substance, *acetanilide* should be used instead of antifebrine.

fibroid, Lat. *fibra* and Gk. εἶδος, "inoid."
fibro'ma, Lat. *fibra* and Gk. -ωμα, inoma.
oros'copy, Lat. *os*, mouth, and Gk. σκοπία,"stomatoscopy."
ovari'tis, Lat. *ovarium* and Gk. ἴτις, oophoritis.
parova'rium, Gk. παρά and Lat. *ovarium*, "paroophorum."
ptæsystol'ic, Lat. *præ* and Gk. συστολικός, "prosystolic."
spec'troscope, Lat. *spectrum* and Gk. σκοπία, "idoscope."
tonsillot'omy, Lat. *tonsilla* and Gk. τομία, amygdalotomy.
tuberculo'sis, Lat. *tuberculum* and Gk.-ωσις,"phymatosis."
uvuli'tis, Lat. *uvula* and Gk. ἴτις, staphylitis or cionitis.
uvulot'omy, Lat. *uvula* and Gk. -τομία, staphylotomy or
    cionotomy.
vaginis'mus, Lat. *vagina* and Gk. -ισμος, colpismus or
    elytrismus.
vagi'nocele, Lat. *vagina* and Gk. κήλη, colpocele.
vulvi'tis, Lat. *vulva* and Gk. -ἴτις, ædœitis feminina.

CHAPTER VIII.

NOMENCLATURE.

NOMENCLATURE is the art of properly arranging and applying a set of distinctive and signfiicant words as the names of particular objects in a science. In botany, for example, it gives the correct names to the various families, genera, and species of plants. Each plant has a *generic* and a *trivial* name, thus in *Spigelia Marilandica*, *Spigelia* designates the genus and *Marilandica* the species of that genus to which the plant belongs. In medical nomenclature no particular system has been adopted. The elementary branches of medical science have required centuries for their development and the numerous hypotheses advanced have all had an influence upon terminology. Even in the naming of diseases and pathological lesions there is no uniformity although various nosologies have been proposed. In anatomy, however, although one of most ancient branches of our science, we find names applied quite systematically, and as anatomical terms are the basis of all nomenclatures in medicine we will devote a few pages to their classification.

I. *Nomenclature of Bones.*

Bones are named (1) from their form or resemblance to some object, (2) from their location, and (3) from some other peculiarity.

1. *Bones with names derived from their form:*

astrag'alus, (ἀστράγαλος, a vertebra); ankle bone.

axis, fr. Greek ἀξών, an axle; second vertebra.

clavic'ulum, dim. of *clavis*, a key; Greek κλείς, root *cleid;* collar bone.

coccyx, Greek κοκκύξ, cuckoo; tail bone.

costæ, Greek πλευραί, from πλευρόν, side; ribs.

fib'ula, Greek περονή, root *perone*, a clasp; brace bone.

il'ium, εἰλεόν, twisted; haunch bone.

incus, fr. *incutio*, to strike; anvil bone.

mal'leus, fr. Aryan *mal*, to strike; hammer bone.

os cuboida'le, κυβοηδής, cube-shaped; cuboid bone.

os cuneifor'me, from *cuneus*, a wedge, and *forma*, shape; cuneiform.

os ethmoida'le, fr. ἠθμωδής, sieve-like; ethmoid.

os hyoi'des, fr. υ, upsilon, and εἶδος, form; *u*-shaped bone.

os magnum, great carpal bone.

os parieta'le, fr. *paries*, a wall; wall bone.

os pisifor'me, fr. *pisis*, a pea, and *forma*, shape; pea-shaped.

os sphenoida'le, σφηνωδής, wedge-shaped; sphenoid.

os scaphoida'le, σκαφωδής, skiff-shaped; scaphoid.

os semiluna're, *semi*, half, *luna*, moon; semilunar.

os turbina'tum, fr. *turba*, a top; top-shaped bone.

os trapezoi'des, τραπεζωδής, table-like; trapezoid.

os uncifor'me, fr. *uncus*, a hook, and *forma*, shape; hook-shaped.

patel'la, dim. of *patina*, a pan; knee pan.

pelvis, Greek πυελός, a basin; pelvis.

phalan'ges, Greek φάλαγγες, batallions; finger bones.

ra'dius, lit. a spoke or ray; forearm bone.

scap'ula, Gk. σκαπαλός, a small shovel; shoulder blade.

sternum, Gk. στέρνον, flat, Sansk. *stirnam;* breast bone.

stapes, allied to *sto*, to stand; stirrup bone.

tib'ia, lit. a flute, Greek κνημη, root *cnem;* shin bone.

trape'zium, fr. τέτρα, four, and ποῦς, a foot, a table; square wrist bone.

vomer, lit. a ploughshare.

2. *Bones with names derived from their location:*

is'chium, Greek ἰσχιός, the haunch; hip bone.

os calca'neum or calcis, fr. *calx*, the heel; heel bone.

os fem'oris, lit. bone of thigh; thigh bone.

os fronta'le or frontis, fr. *frons*, forehead; forehead bone.

os hu'meri, fr. ὦμός, the shoulder; arm bone.

os lachryma'le, fr. *lachryma*, a tear; lachrymal bone.

os mala're, fr. *mala*, cheek; cheek bone.

os maxilla're infe'rius, Gk. μύλον, (root *myl*), a mill.

os maxilla're supe'rius, upper jaw bone.

os nasa'le, fr. *nasus*, nose; nasal bone.

os occipita'le, fr. *occiput*, base of head; occipital bone.

os palata'le, fr. *palatum*, palate; palatal bone.

os pubis, fr. *pubes*, hair, Gk. πεκτήν (*pectin*); pubic bone.

ulna, fr. Greek ὠλένη, elbow; elbow bone.

3. *Miscellaneous:*

Atlas, Greek *Ἄτλας*, the world-supporting giant; first vertebra.

os innomina'tum, fr. *in*, not, *nomino*, to name; unnamed bone.

ossa Wormia'na, fr. *Wormius*, who first described them; Wormian bones.

sacrum, Greek ὀστέον ἅγιον, holy bone; sacred or cursed.

ver'tebra, fr. *verto*, to turn; spindle bone.

II. Nomenclature of Muscles.

Muscles are named (1) from their form, (2) from their action, and (3) from their attachment or location. The names of muscles are used adjectively and are always in the masculine gender agreeing with *musculus* understood.

1. *Form or some peculiarity:*

az'ygos, Greek ἄζυγος, without a fellow.

biceps, *bis* double, *caput* headed.

biven'ter, *bis,* double, *venter,* belly.

complex'us, lit. woven together, fr. *complecto.*

deltoi'deus, Greek δελοιδής, delta (⊿) shaped.

diaphrag'ma, Greek διαφράγμα, a partition.

digas'tricus, Greek δίς, double, γαστήρ, belly.

gemel'lus, dim. of *geminus,* a twin :

    superior, upper.

    inferior, lower.

grac ilis, slender.

latis'simus dorsi, broadest m. of back.

longis'simus dorsi, longest m. of back.

longus colli, long m. of neck.

lumbrica'les, lit. fr. *lumbricus,* a worm ; worm-shaped.

multif'idus spinæ, the m. of the spine split many times.

obliq'uus exter'nus, the external oblique.

obliq'uus internus, the internal oblique.

obtura'tor, *stopper:*

    externus, the external.

    internus, the internal.

orbicula ris oris, circular muscle of mouth.

orbicula'ris palpebra'rum, circular muscle of eyelids.

platys'ma myoi'des, Greek πλάτυσμα μυφδής, the muscle-like expansion.

pyramida'lis, fr. Gk. πυραμίς, a pyramid ; pyramidal.

pyrifor mis, pear-shaped.

quadra'tus, *square:*

    femoris, of thigh.

    lumborum, of loins.

rectus, *straight:*

    abdominis, of abdomen.

    capitis anticus major, larger anterior, of head.

    capitis anticus minor, smaller anterior, of head.

    capitis lateralis, lateral, of head.

    capitis posticus major, larger posterior, of head.

capitis posticus minor, smaller posterior, of head.
   externus, external.
   femoris, of thigh.
   inferior, inferior.
   internus, internal.
   superior, upper.
rhomboi'deus, *rhomb-shaped:*
   major, larger.
   minor, smaller.
scale'nus, *irregular triangular:*
   anticus, anterior.
   medius, middle.
   posticus, posterior.
semimembrano'sus, half membranous.
semitendino'sus, half tendinous.
serra'tus, *toothed:*
   magnus, large.
   posticus inferior, lower posterior.
   posticus superior, upper posterior.
sole'us, sole-shaped, fr. *solea*, a sole or sole fish.
sple'nius, *spleen-shaped:*
   capitis, spleen-shaped, of head.
   colli, spleen-shaped, of neck.
transver'sus perinæ'i, transverse, of perineum.
transversa'lis, *transverse:*
   abdominis, of belly.
   lumborum, of loins.
   cervicis, of neck.
   pedis, of foot.
teres, *round:*
   major, larger.
   minor, smaller.
trape'zius, Greek τράπεζα, a table; table-shaped.
triangula'ris sterni, triangular, of breast-bone.

triceps, three headed, fr. *tris*, triple, and *caput*, head.
vastus, *large:*
> *externus*, external.
> *internus*, internal.

2. *Uses.* Muscles were first classified according to
their function by Galen.
abduc'tor, *leader away:*
> *minimi digiti*, of little finger.
> *pollicis*, of thumb or great toe.

accelera'tor uri'næ, hastener of the urine.
adduc'tor, *leader to:*
> *brevis*, short.
> *longus*, long.
> *magnus*, large.
> *pollicis manus*, of thumb.
> *pollicis pedis*, of great toe.

attol'lens aurem, lifting up the ear.
at'rahens aurem, drawing to the ear.
buccina'tor, trumpeter, because used in inflating cheek.
compres'sor naris, presser together of nostril.
constric'tor ure'thræ, drawer together of urethra.
corruga'tor supercil'ii, wrinkler of eyebrow.
cremas'ter, Greek χρεμαστήρ, the suspender (of testicle).
depres'sor, *presser down:*
> *alæ nasi*, of side of nose.
> *anguli oris*, of corner of mouth.
> *labii inferioris*, of lower lip.

dila'tor naris, expander of nostril.
erec'tor spinæ, straightener of spine.
exten'sor, *extender:*
> *brevis digitorum*, short extender of fingers.
> *carpi radialis brevior*, shorter radial extender of
>   wrist.

carpi radialis longior, longer radial extender of wrist.
carpi ulnaris, ulnar extender of wrist.
communis digitorum, common extender of fingers.
indicis, extender of first finger.
longus digitorum, long extender of fingers.
minimi digiti, extender of little finger.
ossis metacarpi pollicis, extender of metacarpal bone
    of thumb.
proprius pollicis, proper extender of thumb.
primi internodii pollicis, extender of first bone of
    thumb.
secundi internodii pollicis, extender of second bone
    of thumb.

flexor, *bender:*

accessorius, accessory or additional.
brevis digitorum, short, of fingers.
brevis minimi digiti manus, short, of little finger.
brevis minimi digiti pedis, short, of little toe.
brevis pollicis manus, short, of thumb.
brevis pollicis pedis, short, of great toe.
carpi radialis, radial, of wrist.
carpi ulnaris, ulnar, of wrist.
longus digitorum, long, of fingers.
longus pollicis manus, long, of thumb.
longus pollicis pedis, long, of great toe.
profundus digitorum, deep, of fingers.
sublimis digitorum, superficial, of fingers.

leva'tor, *lifter:*

anguli oris, of corner of mouth.
anguli scapulæ, of corner of scapula.
ani et prostatæ, of anus and prostate.
ani et vaginæ, of anus and vagina.
costarum, of ribs.

labii superioris alæque nasi, of upper lip and side of nose.

labii superioris proprius, the proper lifter of upper lip.

menti, of chin.

palati, of palate.

palbebræ superioris, of upper eyelid.

masse′ter, Greek μασσητήρ, the masticator, chewer.

oppo′nens, *opposing:*

minimi digiti, of little finger.

pollicis, of thumb.

prona′tor, *turner downward:*

quadratus, square.

radii teres, round, of radius.

ret′rahens aurem, drawing back the ear.

riso′rius, the laughing muscle, fr. *rideo,* to laugh.

sarto′rius, the tailor muscle, fr. *sartor,* a tailor, because used in crossing the legs as tailors do.

sphincter, *drawer together,* fr. σφίγγω, to tie up a bag:

ani externus, external compressor of anus.

ani internus, internal compressor of anus.

vaginæ, compressor of vagina.

tensor, *stretcher:*

palati, of palate.

vaginæ femoris, of sheath of thigh.

3. *Location and attachment:*

ancone′us, fr. Greek ἀγκών, the elbow; elbow muscle.

arytenoi′deus, Gk. ἀρυτενοειδής, pitcher-like; attached to arytenoid cartilage.

brachia′lis anti′cus, anterior arm.

cervica′lis ascen′dens, ascending neck.

coccyge′us, coccygeal muscle.

cor′aco-brachia′lis, attached to coracoid process and arm.

crico-thyroi′deus, attached to cricoid and thyroid cartilages.

crure'us, leg muscle, fr. *crus,* the leg.

gastrocne'mius, calf of leg m., fr. γαστήρ, belly, and κνήμη, leg.

genio-hyo-glos'sus, (Gk. γενεῖο-ὑο-γλῶσσα) attached to chin, hyoid, and tongue.

genio-hyoid'eus, Gk. γενεῖον and ὑοιδής, attached to chin and hyoid.

glute'us, fr. Greek γλουτοί, *buttocks:*
    maximus, largest buttock.
    medius, middle buttock.
    minimus, smallest buttock.

hyo-glos'sus, Gk. ὑοιδής and γλῶσσα, attached to hyoid and tongue.

ili'acus, iliac muscle, fr. *ilium,* haunch bone.

infraspina'tus, below the spine (of scapula).

intercosta'les, *between the ribs:*
    externi, external.
    interni, internal.

supina'tor, *layer on the back:*
    brevis, short.
    longus, long.

interos'sei manus vel pedis, between the bones of hand or foot.

interspina'les, between the spines of the vertebræ.

intertransversa'les, between the transverse processes of vertebræ.

is'chio-caverno'sus, attached to ischium and corpus cavernosum.

mylo-hyoi'deus, Greek μύλον, lower jaw; attached to lower jaw and hyoid.

occip'ito-fronta'lis, attached to occiput and frontal bone.

omo-hyoi'deus, Greek ὦμος, shoulder; attached to shoulder and hyoid.

19

palma'ris, *palmar:*
> *brevis,* short.
> *longus,* long.

pala'to-glos'sus, attached to palate and tongue.

pala'to-pharyn'geus, attached to palate and pharynx.

pectine'us, Greek πεκτήν, the pubic bone; attached to pubic bone.

pectora'lis, *belonging to chest:*
> *major,* greater chest muscle.
> *minor,* lesser chest muscle.

perone'us, *fibular,* fr. περόνη, fibula:
> *brevis,* short.
> *longus,* long.
> *tertius,* third.

planta'ris, belonging to sole (*planta*) of foot.

poplite'us, located near *poplites* or ham-strings.

psoas (Greek ψωά) *the loin:*
> *magnus,* large.
> *parvus,* small.

pterygoi'deus:
> *externus,* attached outside of pterygoid process.
> *internus,* attached inside of pterygoid process.

sacro-lumba'lis, attached to sacrum and loin.

salpin'go-pharyn'geus, attached to Eustachian tube and pharynx.

semispina'lis, *attached half to spine:*
> *colli,* of neck.
> *dorsi,* of back.

spina'lis dorsi, attached to spine of back.

sterno-cleido-mastoi'deus, attached to breast bone, clavicle, and mastoid process of temporal bone

sterno-hyoi'deus, attached to sternum and hyoid.

sterno-thyroi'deus, attached to sternum and thyroid cartilage.

stylo-glos'sus, attached to styloid process and tongue.
stylo-hyoi'deus, attached to styloid process and hyoid bone.
stylo-pharyn'geus, attached to styloid process and pharynx.
subcla'vius, located under the clavicle.
subcrure'us, located under the crureus muscle.
subscapula'ris, located under the scapula.
supraspina'tus, located over the spine of scapula.
tempora'lis, attached to temporal region.
thyro-arytenoi'deus, attached to thyroid and arytenoid cartilages.
thyro-hyoi'deus, attached to thyroid cartilage and hyoid bone.
tibia'lis, *attached to tibia:*
  anticus, attached to tibia in front.
  posticus, attached to tibia behind.
trache'lo-mastoi'deus, attached to neck and mastoid process.
zygomat'icus, *attached to zygoma:*
  major, greater.
  minor, lesser.

III. *Nomenclature of Arteries.*

Arteries are named (1) from their location, (2) from the parts which they supply, and (3) from some peculiarity in their form or position.

The names of arteries are always feminine agreeing with *arteria* expressed or understood.

1. *Location:*

axilla'ris, located in axilla.
axis cœli'aca, belly axis of arteries.
basila'ris, located on basilar process of occipital bone.
perone'al, fibular.

sciat'ica, fr. ἰσχιατική, the haunch or thigh.
subscla'vian, under the clavicle.
submenta'lis, under the chin.
superficia'lis volæ, superficial of palm, *vola.*

2. *Parts supplied:*

alveola'ris, supplying tooth sockets, *alveoli.*
bucca'lis, supplying mouth, *bucca.*
cys'tica, supplying gall bladder.
gas'trica, supplying stomach.
hemorrhoida'lis, supplying the hemorrhoids of rectum.
hepat'ica, supplying liver.
phren'ica, supplying diaphragm (φρήν.)
pu'dica, supplying *pudenda* or genitals.
rani'na, supplying *rana* or tip of tongue; lit. the *frog.*

3. *Miscellaneous:*

aor'ta, Greek ἀωρτή, from ἀείρω, to rise up.
anastomat'ica, anastomosing, inosculating.
corona'ria, surrounding mouth or heart like a crown,
corona.
carot'ida, fr. Gk. καρόω, to throttle, fr. κάρα, to head.
circum'flex, bending around, fr. *circumfligo.*
innomina'ta, located in a place unnamed and supplying
no particular part.
recur'rens, running back.

IV. *Nomenclature of veins.*

The names of veins are formed in the same manner
as those of arteries and are likewise feminine, agreeing
with *vena,* expressed or understood. In the majority of
cases the names of the veins are identical with those of
the arteries in the same location. We give below the
names of veins derived from some peculiarity:

fasil'ica, fr. βασιλικός, royal; large.
cava, hollow, because usually found empty after death.
cephal'ica, because opened in diseases of the head.
jugula'ris, fr. *jugulum,* a name for throat; fr. *jugum,* a yoke.
saphe'na, Gk. σαφηνής, clear; manifest; because easily seen through skin.
venæ com'ites, companion veins, because accompanying arteries.
venæ Gale'ni, veins of Galen because discovered by him.
vena portæ, the vein of the *gate* of liver.

V. Nomenclature of Nerves.

Nerves are named (1) from their function, (2) from their location, (3) from the parts which they supply, and (4) from some peculiarity. The names of nerves are always masculine agreeing with *nervus* expressed or understood. We give examples of each method of formation.

1. Function:

audito'rius, fr. *audio,* to hear; the hearing nerve.
gustato'rius, fr. *gusto,* to taste; the tasting nerve.
op'ticus, fr. Greek ὄπτω, to see; the seeing nerve.
olfacto'rius, fr. *olfacere,* to smell; the smelling nerve.
pathet'icus, fr. Gk. πάθος, feeling; the nerve which expresses the feelings by the eye.
sympathet'icus, the harmonizing nerve (συμπάθομαι, to feel together).

2. Location:

auricula'ris, belonging to ear.
facia'lis, belonging to, also supplying face.
hypoglossa'lis, located under (ὑπό) the tongue (γλῶσσα).
media'nus, the middle nerve of arm, fr. *medius,* middle.

menta'lis, located on chin (*mentum*).
sciat'icus, located on thigh or haunch (*ἰσχίον*).

3. *Part supplied:*

abdu'cens, supplying external rectus; abductor of eye.
glosso-pharyngea'lis, supplying tongue and pharynx.
genito-crura'lis, supplying genitals and leg.
musculo-cuta'neus, supplying muscles and skin.
pneumo-gas'tricus, supplying air-passages and stomach.
trochlea'ris, supplying the trochlear or superior oblique
    muscle.

4. *Miscellaneous:*

descen'dens noni, descending branch of ninth cranial.
mus'culo-spira'lis, twisting around downward and sup-
    plying muscles.
por'tio mollis sep'timi, soft part of seventh, auditory.
por'tio dura sep'timi, hard part of seventh, facial.
trigem'inus, triple, from *trigemini*, triplets.
Vidia'nus, named in honor of *Vidius*, an Italian anatomist.

VI. *Encephalogical Nomenclature.*

In naming the parts of the brain no system has
been adopted. The earlier anatomists believed that in
the brain could be found the homologues of all the other
parts of the body and this hypothesis has had a great
influence upon the nomenclature. Other parts have been
named from a fancied resemblance to some familiar
object.

amyg'dala, Greek *ἀμυγδάλη*, an almond; a tonsil.
aqueduc'tus Syl'vii, conduit of Sylvius.
arach'noid, Greek *ἀραχνοειδής*, like a spider web.
arbor vitæ, tree of life.
bra'chium, Greek *βραχίων*, an arm.
cal'amus scriptori'us, Greek *κάλαμος*, a reed, writing pen.

cap'sula, dim. of *capsa*, a box.
centrum majus, larger center.
centrum minus, smaller center.
centrum ova le, oval center.
claustrum, a barrier, a sheet.
clava, a club, a penis.
cer'ebrum, the brain, cf. *κάρα*, the head.
crebel lum, dim. of *cerebrum*.
choroid plexus, leather-like net work.
cor'nua, horns.
commissu'ra, a joining together.
corpus denta'tum, toothed body.
corpus callo'sum, callous body.
corpus fimbria'tum, fringed body.
corpus stria'tum, striped body.
cor'pora genicula'ta, knee-like or bent bodies.
cor'pora mammilla'ria, breast-like bodies.
cor'pora quadrigem'ina, quadruplet bodies.
crura cer'ebri, legs of brain.
dura mater, hard mother or membrane.
fissu'ræ, clefts.
floc'culus, a tuft of wool.
fornix, an arch; union, connection.
funic'ulus, a small cord.
falx cer'ebri, sickle of brain.
genu, knee.
hippocam'pus, Greek *ἱπποκάμπος*, a sea animal with a horse's head.
infundib'ulum, a small funnel.
iter e tertio ad quartum ventric'ulum, passage from the third to the fourth ventricles.
lin'gula, small tongue.
lam'ina cine'ria, ash-colored layer.
lobus quadra'tus, square lobe.

nates, buttocks.

nodule, small knot.

nu'cleus cauda'tus, tailed kernel.

nu'cleus lenticula'ris, lentil-like kernel.

pedun'cula, little feet.

pia mater, tender mother or membrane.

pyram'idal body or **lobe,** pyramid-shaped body.

pin'eal gland, shaped like a pine cone.

pitu'itary body, mucus secreting body.

proces'sus e cerebello ad testes, process from small
        brain to testicles of brain.

pons Varo'lii, the bridge of Varolius.

raphe, a seam.

rostrum, a beak or prow.

rest'iform body, rope-like body.

septum lu'cidum, transparent partition.

sple'nium, spleen.

striæ acus'ticæ (Gk. ἀκουστικαί) auditory stripes.

tæ'nia semicircula'ris, semicircular ribbon.

testes, testicles.

thal'amus (Greek θάλαμός) a marriage bed.

tuber cine'reum, ashy protuberance.

tento'rium, a tent.

u'vula, a small grape, the uvula.

velum interpos'itum, the interposed veil.

vallec'ula, small valley.

ven'tricles, small stomachs.

vulva cere'bri, vulva of brain.

PART IV

ELEMENTS DERIVED FROM THE MODERN LANGUAGES.

CHAPTER I.

THE FRENCH ELEMENT.

THE great majority of the foreign words found in our medical books are of French origin. Many of these words have been modified in form and have become essentially English words, both in appearance and pronunciation. For example, *dartrous*, a word applied to a diathesis in which there is a tendency to skin disease, is derived from the French *dartre*, from the Greek δείρω, to flay, or δαρτός, flayed. But besides these Anglicised French words, there are numerous examples of real foreigners in our language, and it is customary with scholars to pronounce these as they are pronounced in their native land. The first French words which found their way into English medical literature were terms applied to venereal diseases and obstetrics; then came the nomenclature of auscultation, which was adopted almost without alteration, and recently a number of neurological terms have been introduced.

The proper pronunciation of French words is a very difficult matter for English-speaking people. The nasal sounds are different from anything in our language. If you will pronounce our nasal *ng*, omitting the final hard *g* sound, you will have a sound very much like the French nasal. There are four of these nasal sounds in French, which may be indicated as follows: —

an, am, em and en, all pronounced *ŏng*, somewhat as in swän(g).

om and on, pronounced *ŏng*, somewhat as in dōn(g).

im, in, aim, ain, ien, yen, pronounced *äng*, somewhat as in an(g)ry.

um and un, pronounced *ŭng*, somewhat as in bun(g).

The French *u* is pronounced like the German *ü* (*ue*), there being no similar sound in English. *G* soft and *j* are pronounced like *z* in azure or *s* in pleasure.

There is no such thing as accent, as we use the term, in the French language; syllables all have nearly the same stress of voice. English speakers erroneously place an accent on the last syllable of French words.

In the following list of words we indicate the pronunciation by the ordinary sounds of English letters, designating the nasals by *ŏng, ŏng, äng* and *ŭng*. In cases where the French pronunciation has been abandoned, this fact will be indicated by (Angl.) placed after the word.

ague (Angl.), originally acute fever, fr. Lat. *acutus*, sharp; sudden.

absinthe (äb-sängt), a cordial containing wormwood, *absinthium.*

accoucheur (äc-cōō-shūr), an obstetrician; a noun derived fr. *accoucher*, fr. Lat. *ad collocare*, which meant to go to bed; since the 13th century used for going into child-bed.

ballottement (bäl-lŏt-mŏng), fr. *ballotter*, to toss a ball, a term first used in tennis playing. Ballottement means, like the tossing of a ball, the fœtus bounding in the amniotic fluid.

bougie (bōō-zhē), lit. a wax candle made in *Bougie*, Algeria. A candle-like instrument or medicated cylinder to be introduced into cavities.

bougie a boule (bōō-zhē ä bōōl), a ball tipped bougie, fr. Latin *bulla*, a ball.

bredouillement (brĕd-ōō-ē-yĕ-mŏng), fr. *bredouiller*, to stammer. Very rapid speech.

bruit (brwē), a roaring noise, fr. Lat. *rugio*, to roar; a sound heard in auscultation.

bruit de craquement (brwē dē crăk-mŏng), a crackling sound.

bruit de cuir neuf (brwē dē quēr nūf), new leather sound.

bruit de diable (brwē de de-äbl), devil's sound, applied to a musical murmur heard in anæmia.

bruit de pot file (brwē de pō fē-lä), cracked-pot sound.

bruit de clapottement (brwē de clä-pŏt-mŏng), swashing sound.

bouillon (bōō-ē-yōng), broth fr. *bouiller*, to boil, Lat. *bullire*.

burette (bū-rĕt), a cruet, a chemical instrument.

bruit de souffle (brwē de sōōfl), bellows sound.

bruit tympanique (brwē tĕm-păn-ēēk), drum sound.

bubon d'emblee (bwē-bōng dŏng-blä), "bubo of onset," applied to buboes which precede the venereal disease.

centigrade (sŏng-tē-grăd), the name of a thermometric scale, fr. *centum*, 100 and *gradum*, step.

chancre Fr. (shŏngkr) (Angl. shänker), a venereal sore, fr. Lat. *cancer*.

chordee (kōr-dä) fr. Lat. *chordatus*, corded, twisted.

clairvoyance (clär-voy-yŏngs) lit. clear vision, "second sight."

clinique (klin-ēēk) lit. clinical, at the bedside; a lecture at the bedside.

conduit Angl. (cŏn-dīt), fr. Lat. *conductus*, conductor pipe.

consomme (kōng-sŏm-mä), fr. Lat. *consummatus*, complete; a thickened soup.

contre coup (cŏngtr kōō), fr. Lat. *contra colpum*, against the blow, applied to injuries on opposite side of head from place where blow was received.

coup de soleil (kōō de sō-lä-yŭh), Lat. *colpus de sole*, stroke from the sun, sun-stroke.

craquement pulmonaire (krăk-mŏng puel-mōn-är), pulmonary crackling sound.

condom (Angl. kŏn-dŏm), fr. the name of the inventor Dr Condom, a membranous cover for penis.

chariere filiere (shär-i-är fĕl-i-är), Chariere's scale of urethral sounds.   French scale.

charbon (shär-bōng), fr. Latin *carbo*, charcoal; *anthrax*.

curette (cuer-et), fr. *curer*, to clean; a scraper.

charpie (shär-pē), fr. Latin *carpere*, to pick; picked lint.

coup de sang (kōō de sŏng), blood stroke; apoplexy.

coup de vent (kōō de vŏng), wind stroke; sudden cold from exposure to wind.

couveuse (cōō-veuz), fr. *couver*, to hatch; an apparatus for rearing children prematurely born.

cul de sac (cuel de săc), bottom of a bag, blind pouch; fr. Lat *collum de sacco*, neck of a bag.

choc en retour (shŏck ŏng r'tōōr), return shock; a term applied to the infection of the mother by a syphilitic fœtus *in utero*.

debris (d'brēē), from *débriser*, to break down; *detritus*.

douche (dōōsh), fr. Italian *doccio*, a shower bath; a wash by means of a tube; an irrigation.

dragee (drä-zhä), lit. a sugar plum; a coated pill.

ecraseur (ĕc-rä-zeur), from *ecraser*, to rub out; an instrument for crushing off a part.

embonpoint (ŏng-bōng-pwŏng), fr. Latin *in bono puncto*, in good condition; plumpness.

enceinte (ŏng-sänt), fr. Latin *incincta*, girded up, pregnant

ergot (Angl.), lit. a spur of a bird; spurred rye.

folie a deux (fōlĕ ä dẽu), insanity of two in same family; quasi-infectious insanity.

folie circulaire (fō-lĕ sir-kue-lär), circular insanity; insanity with mania, melancholy, stupor and lucidity following regularly and repeatedly.

fontenelle (fōngt-nĕl), fr. Latin *fontenella*, a little fountain; the soft part, not covered with bone, of an infant's head.

fourchette (fōōr-shĕt), dim. of *fourche*, Lat. *forcus*, a fork.

gavage (gä-väzh), fr. *gaver*, to stuff; forced alimentation.

goitre (Angl. goyter), fr. Latin *guttur*, the throat; enlargement of thyroid gland.

gorget (Angl.), fr. old French word meaning throat, *gorge*, from Latin *gurges*, a whirlpool; now applied to a beaked knife.

grand mal (grŏng mäl), great sickness; *epilepsia gravior*.

jaundice (Angl.), fr. *jaunisse*, yellowness of skin.

lavage (lä-väzh), fr. *laver*, to wash; washing of cavities, especially the stomach.

mal de mer (mäl dĕ mär), sea sickness.

manie sans delire (mänĕ sŏng delĕr), insanity without delirium; emotional insanity.

massage (mäs-säzh), from *masser*, to rub; treatment by shampooing and rubbing.

masseur (m) (mäs-seūr), } one who practices massage.
masseuse (f) (mäs-seuz), }

mayhem, Old French word meaning disfiguring.

main en griffe (mäng ŏng grĕf), clawed hand; a symptom in some nervous affections.

muguet (mue-gwä), fr. *muscus*, musk; thrush.

panaris (pän-är-ē), fr. Latin *panaricium*, a whitlow; now syphilitic disease of fingers; dactylitis.

pomegranate, (Angl.) fr. *pome*, apple, and *granate*, seeded.

perleche (pär-lĕsh), fr. *perlecher*, to lick; a contagious disease of the mouth.

petit mal (p'tē mǎl), small sickness, *epilepsia mitior.*

physique (fīz-ēēk), fr. φυσικός, natural; the natural form.

rale (rŏl), fr. *raler*, to rattle; a rattling, *rhonchus.*

rale crepitant (rŏl crä-pē-tŏng), a crackling rattle.

rale muqueuse (rŏl mü-keūz), a mucous rattle.

rale sibilant (rŏl sē-bē-lŏng), a whistling rattle.

rale sonore (rŏl sō-nōre), snoring rattle.

serre fine (sär fēēn), lit. fine teeth of a saw; a catch pin.

souffle (sōōfl), a breathing or bellows sound, fr. Latin *sufflare*, to blow up.

tache cerebrale (täsh sär-e-brǎl), cerebral touch; an irritable condition of skin observed in nervous diseases.

tampon (tŏng-pōng), a plug, for vagina.

tic douloureux (tēēk dōō-lōō-reū), painful fit; trigeminal neuralgia.

tourniquet (Angl. tour-nīkĕt), fr. *tourner*, to turn, a turnstile; an instrument for compressing arteries.

trigone (trē-gōn), fr. Gk. τριγωνία, a triangle; triangular space of bladder.

trocar (Angl.), fr. *trois quarts* (trwä kär) three cornered; from the shape of the instrument.

THE METRIC SYSTEM.

The metric system of weights and measures first employed in France has been adopted by scientists throughout the world, and attempts have recently been made to have it adopted in dispensing and prescription writing.

The unit of the metric system is the *metre* (mātr), supposed to equal $\frac{1}{10000000}$ of the distance from the Equator to the Pole, or about 39.37 inches. The word *metre* is derived from the Greek μέτρον, a measure. The *metre* is strictly the unit of measures of length.

Fractional parts of the unit are expressed by pre-fixing the Latin *decimals, decem, centum* and *mille* to the unit. *Multiples* are derived from the Greek decimals, δέχα, ἑκατόν, χίλιος and μύριος.

The fractionals are abbreviated by taking the first letter of the decimal in small type and the first letter of the unit. The multiples are abbreviated by taking the Roman capital equivalent of the first letter of the Greek decimal and the small first letter of the unit.

The cube of a tenth part of a metre is taken as the unit of measures of capacity. This is called a *litre* (lētr), and is equal to about thirty-four fluid ounces. The word *litre* is derived from the Greek λίτρα, a weight equal to about twelve ounces avoirdupois.

The weight of a thousandth part of a litre of water at its maximum density (4 deg. C.) is taken as the unit of measures of weight and is called a *gramme* (grăm.), from the Greek γράμμα, a weight equal to the Latin *scrupulus* or $\frac{1}{24}$ of an ounce. A cubic centimetre of water at its maximum density also weighs one gramme.

From these units the following tables have been constructed:—

I. *Measures of Length.*

Fractionals :

Millimetre (mm.) $= \frac{metre}{1000} =$ .039$\frac{1}{3}$ in., nearly $\frac{1}{25}$ of an inch.

Centimetre (cm.) $= \frac{metre}{100} =$ .3937 in., nearly $\frac{2}{5}$ of an inch.

Decimeter (dm.) $= \frac{metre}{10} =$ 3.937 in., nearly 4 inches.

Unit:

Metre (m.) $=$ 39.37 in. about 3$\frac{1}{4}$ ft.

Multiples :

Decametre (Dm.) $=$ metre $\times$ 10 $=$ about 33 ft.

Hectometre (Hm.) $=$ metre $\times$ 100 $=$ about 328 ft.

Kilometre (Km.) $=$ metre $\times$ 1000 $=$ about $\frac{3}{5}$ of a mile.

Myriametre (Mm.) $=$ metre $\times$ 10000 $=$ about 6$\frac{1}{5}$ miles.

The French word *metre* is now often Anglicised as *meter* and the numeral prefixes are pronounced as if they were pure English; thus, mĭl lĭ mē-ter instead of mēel-mātr, sĕn-tĭ-mē-ter instead of sŏng-tē-mātr, etc.   Since these words are so commonly used and so generally mispronounced as spelled in French, it is probably better to pronounce and spell them according to English methods.

II.   *Measures of Capacity.*

Fractionals:

Millilitre (ml. or cc. $_{\text{centimetre}}^{\text{for cu.}}$) $= \frac{\text{litre}}{1000} =$ about 16 minims.

Centilitre (cl.) $= \frac{\text{litre}}{100} = f\,\mathrec{3}$ij. ℳxl. nearly.

Decilitre (dl.) $= \frac{\text{litre}}{10} = f\,\mathrm{3}$iij. ℥iij. nearly.

UNIT:

Litre   (l.) $=$ O. ij. ℥ij. nearly.

Multiples:

Decalitre (Dl.) $=$ l. × 10 $=$ O. xxi. ℥iij.

Hectolitre (Hl.) $=$ l. × 100 $=$ C. xxvi.

Kilolitre (Kl.) $=$ l. × 1000 $=$ about 8 bbls.

III.   *Measures of Weight.*

Fractionals:

Milligramme (mg.) $= \frac{\text{gramme}}{1000} =$ gr. $\frac{1}{66}$ nearly.

Centigramme (cg.) $= \frac{\text{gramme}}{100} =$ gr. $\frac{2}{13}$ nearly.

Decigramme   (dg.) $= \frac{\text{gramme}}{10} =$ gr. iss. nearly.

UNIT:
Gramme   (Gm.) $=$ gr. xvss. nearly.

Multiples:

Decagramme (Dg.) $=$ Gm. × 10 $=$ ℥ij. gr. xxxiv. nearly

Hectogramme (Hg.) $=$ Gm. × 100 $=$ ℥iij. ℥iss.

Kilogramme (Kg.) $=$ Gm. × 1000 $=$ lb. ijss. nearly.

Myriagramme (Mg.) $=$ Gm. × 10000 $=$ 27 ℔s. nearly.

The units of the measures of capacity and weight are now often spelled *liter* and *gram*, and all fractional multiples are pronounced as if they were English words.

CHAPTER II.

Words Derived from Other Modern Languages.

I. *Words derived from the Italian.*

A few Italian words have found their way into the English medical vocabulary. Many of these are so much like Latin words that they are commonly treated as such, yet they come indirectly from the Latin through the Italian. It is not customary to give these words the Italian pronunciation as they have become naturalized in our language and are really English words of Italian origin.

belladon'na, fr. *bella*, beautiful, and *donna*, lady, so called because used to dilate the pupils and give the eyes a bright appearance.

ber'gamot, fr. Italian *bergamotto*, a pear.

bun'ion, fr. Italian *bugnone*, a lump, allied to Scandinavian *bunki*, a bunch. Thomas derives bunion from the Greek βούνιον, a peanut.

cel'ery, fr Italian *seleri*, fr. Greek σέλινον, parsley.

influen'za, lit. *influence*, or *flowing upon;* epidemic coryza.

Lazaret'to, plural *Lazaretti*, a pest-house, fr. the New Testament beggar, *Lazarus*.

mala'ria, fr. *mala*, bad, and *aria*, air or appearance; *mal' aria*, Latin *malus ær*, a miasm.

rube'ola, lit. "a little red berry," from the color of the spots, measles.

rose'ola, from Italian *rosiola*, measles, dim. of *rosa*, a rose; rose rash.

scarlati'na, fr. Italian *scarlattina*, from Persian *saqalat*, scarlet; scarlet fever.

seton, from Italian *setone*, a horse hair, of which setons were first made.

soda, an ash used in making glass, fr. Lat. *solida*, solid.

trepan, fr. Italian *trepano*, a turnstile, from Greek τρέπω, to turn.

II. *Words derived from the Spanish.*

The Spanish words found in medical works are generally the names of medicinal plants. They are pronounced and treated as Latin words.

Angustu'ra, a bitter plant from Angostura, a city of Venezuela.

calisa'ya, a name for yellow Peruvian bark.

ca'cao, fr. the Mexican name of the chocolate tree.

cas'cara sagra'da, lit. sacred bark; buckthorn.

cascaril'la, dim. of *cascara*, little bark; jesuits' bark.

copai'ba, fr. *copal*, a fragrant gum and *iba*, tree.

coch'ineal, fr. Spanish *cochinella*, dim. of Greek κόκκος, a berry, little berries, which they resemble.

damia'na, a fanciful derivation is "Dami Anna," "Give me Anna," a notorious prostitute in the town where this plant was first used as an aphrodisiac.

dengue (dăng-ga), lit. a short veil, so called because the eyes are sometimes affected in this disease as if a veil were thrown over them; breakbone fever.

hedeo'ma, fr. *heder*, to be odorous; pennyroyal.

guai'acum, fr. Sp. *guaiaco*, lignum vitæ.

guano, fr. Peruvian *huano*, dung.

jalap, fr. Sp. *Xalapa*, a town in Mexico.

manzani'ta, dim. of *manzana*, apple; crab apple.

plat'inum, fr. Sp. *plata*, silver.

sherry, fr. *Xeres*, a town in Spain from which this wine was exported.

sarsaparil'la, fr. Sp. *zarzarparilla,* "a little prickly vine," smilax.

vanil'la, fr. Sp. *vainilla,* a small sheath or pod; Latin *vaginella.*

yerba buena, "good plant;" micromeria.

yerba santa, holy herb, fr. Lat. *herba sancta*; eriodictyon.

Xer'icum, fr. *Xeres,* cf. sherry.

III. Words of Portuguese Origin.

The Portuguese words found in medical works have in most instances come from South America. They are in their turn often derived from native Indian words.

cincho'na, named after the Countess of Cinchon; Peruvian bark.

guara'na, Paraguay tea; maté.

mona'ca, bone *manar,* to distil from, because it is supposed to distil disease from the system.

jaboran'di (zhäböröndë), pilocarpus.

porten'se, fr. *Oporto,* a city of Portugal.

pimen'ta, allspice, lit. a dark spiced drink, fr. Latin *pigmentum,* paint.

IV. Words of German origin.

Baunsheidt'ismus, fr. Dr. Baunsheidt, who invented this method of counter-irritation.

bismuth, fr. *wiszmuth,* "white mind," a metal.

cobalt, fr. *kobald,* a goblin; a metal.

Mes'merism, from *Mesmer,* the discoverer of the phenomenon.

rin'derpest, cattle plague.

rœtheln, dim. of *roth,* red; German measles.

zinc, allied to *zinn,* tin; a tin-like metal.

V. Words of Dutch origin.

litmus, fr. *lackmus,* a dyestuff.

man'ikin, dim. of man.

measles, dim. of *masa,* a spot.

mumps, fr. *mompen,* to sulk.

scalp, fr. *scalpe,* the scalp.

17.   Words of Scandinavian origin.

radezyge (räh'de-zēgüh), lit. scab sickness; Norwegian leprosy.

skull, fr. Danish *skaal,* a basin.

thrush, fr. Icelandic *thurrish,* dryish; muguet.

tungsten, Swedish *tung,* heavy, and *sten,* stone; a metal.

Yt'trium, fr. *Ytterby,* a town in Sweden; a metal.

GENERAL INDEX.

INDEX OF WORDS.

fomes, 147.
fons, 147.
fontenelle, 291.
foramen, 114.
forma, 97.
formica, 45.
formula, 97.
fornix, 153.
fortior, 152.
fourchette, 291.
frænum, 150.
fragrans, 149.
frangula, 97.
frigus, 153.
frons, 153.
fructus, 122.
frumentum, 134.
fulcrum, 150.
fulvus, 153.
fundus, 103.
funiculus, 103.
funis, 112.
furfur, 108.
fusus, 153.

G.

galactæmia, 232.
galactagogue, 233.
galactorrhœa, 255.
galactosuria, 261.
galacturia, 261.
galla, 97.
gallicus, 153.
gallus, 165.
galvanism, 41.
ganboge, 41.
ganglion, 104.
gangrene, 264.
gas, 45.
gastralgia, 234.
gastricus, 153.
gastritis, 241.
gastrocele, 236.
gastrodynia, 246.
gastrology, 246.
gastroplasty, 253.
gastrorrhœa, 255.
gastroscopy, 258.
gaultheria, 97.
gavage, 291.
gelsemium, 150.
geminus, 153.
gemma, 95.

gena, 97.
gentian, 4.
genu, 124.
genus, 153.
glaber, 139.
gladiolus, 103.
glandula, 97.
glans, 154.
glaucus, 153.
glenoid, 248.
glioma, 249.
globus, 103.
glossalgia, 234.
glossectomy, 237.
glossitis, 241.
glossology, 243.
glottis, 118.
gluten, 154.
glycosuria, 261.
gnathoplasty, 253.
god, 44.
goitre, 291.
gomphosis, 256.
gonagra, 234.
gonocace, 236.
gonorrhœa, 47.
gorget, 291.
gossypium, 150.
gracilis, 164.
gramen, 114.
grand mal, 291.
granum, 150.
graphite, 264.
-graphy, 238.
gratus, 153.
gravidus, 153.
gravis, 164.
guano, 296.
guaiacum, 296.
guarana, 297.
gubernaculum, 131.
guillotine, 41.
gustus, 122.
gutta, 95.
gutta percha, 32.
gynæcology, 243.
gynæcoscopy, 258.
gynatresia, 235.

H.

habit, 103.
habitus, 122.
hæmaglobinuria, 261.

hæmatocele, 236.
hæmatemesis, 256.
hæmatoid, 245.
hæmatoma, 248.
hæmatopsia, 251.
hæmatoxylon, 104.
hæmaturia, 261.
hæmology, 243.
hæmoptysis, 264.
hæmorrhagia, 254.
halitus, 122.
hallux, 187.
halo, 154.
halogen, 264.
halloid, 245.
hamamelis, 118.
haustus, 122.
heal, 25.
hectic, 264.
hedeoma, 296.
helcoid, 248.
helcoplasty, 253.
helcosis, 256.
helix, 154.
helminthiasis, 256.
helminthology, 243.
hemeralopia, 251.
hemianæsthesia, 224.
hemianopsia, 224.
hemichorea, 224.
hemicrania, 224.
hemiopia, 224.
hemiplegia, 224.
hemisphere, 224.
hepar, 119.
hepaticus, 155.
hepatitis, 241.
hepatocele, 236.
hepatoncus, 250.
herbarium, 134.
heri, 179.
hermaphrodite, 50.
hernia, 264.
heroic, 239.
herpes, 264.
hic, 167.
hilum, 142.
hippus, 264.
hirudo, 154.
histology, 243.
histolysis, 256.
homo, 39, 150.
homœopathy, 252.

metralgia, 234.
metria, 239.
metritis, 241.
metrodynia, 246.
metrorrhagia, 254.
metrorrhœa, 255.
miasma, 265.
microbiology, 244.
micrococcus, 265.
micropsia, 251.
microscopy, 258.
migraine, 50.
molaris, 164.
molimen, 114.
mollities, 126.
molluscum, 165.
momentum, 165.
monaco, 297.
monad, 230.
monandrous, 230.
monograph, 230.
monomania, 230.
monobasic, 230.
monorchis, 230.
mons, 168.
monstrum, 165.
morbidus, 164.
morphine, 4.
morphology, 244.
morrhua, 99.
mors, 145.
morsus, 181.
mortalis, 164.
moschus, 11.
motus, 122.
mucilago, 168.
muguet, 291.
muliebris, 160.
multus, 155.
mumps, 298.
musculus, 105.
myalgia, 234.
myelitis, 241.
myelomalacia, 245.
myograph, 238.
myoid, 248.
myology, 241.
myoma, 250.
myopia, 251.
myositis, 241.
mysophobia, 252.
myxœdema, 247.
myxology, 244.

myxoma, 250.

N.

nævus, 105.
nanoid, 248.
nanus, 105.
naphtha, 29.
nard, 31.
naris, 112.
nasturtium, 156.
nasus, 156.
natura, 101.
nausea, 40.
nebula, 101.
nec, 187.
necrology, 244.
necrosis, 257.
nematoid, 248.
nephralgia, 235.
nephrectomy, 237.
nephritis, 241.
nephrology, 244.
nephroid, 248.
nephrotomy, 260.
nervus, 105.
neuralgia, 235.
neurectomy, 237.
neurilemma, 265.
neuritis, 241.
neurology, 244.
neuroma, 250.
neuroglia, 265.
neuropathy, 252.
neurorrhaphy, 253.
neurotomy, 260.
neuter, 141.

O.

obliquus, 164.
occidentalis, 160.
occiput, 169.
octarius, 110.
oculus, 110.
odontalgia, 235.
odontagra, 234.
odontoid, 248.
odontoma, 250.
odontology, 244.
-odynia, 246.
-œdema, 246.
œnomania, 246.
œsophagismus, 259.
œsophagitis, 241.

œsophagotomy, 260.
officina, 101.
-oid, 247.
olecranon, 265.
oleum, 165.
olfactus, 122.
oleoresina, 101.
olighæmia, 233.
oliguria, 261.
omagra, 234.
omentum, 134.
oncology, 244.
-oncus, 250.
onychia, 239.
oöphoralgia, 235.
oöphoritis, 241.
oöphorectomy, 237.
opacus, 160.
ophthalmagra, 234.
ophthalmectomy, 237.
ophthalmia, 239.
ophthalmitis, 241.
ophthalmodynia, 246.
ophthalmology, 244.
ophthalmorrhœa, 255.
ophthalmoscopy, 258.
opium, 178.
opponens, 149.
opticus, 160.
orange, 31.
orbicularis, 169.
orbita, 101.
orchialgia, 235.
orchiectomy, 237.
orchitis, 241.
orchiotomy, 260.
organum, 159.
origo, 174.
oroscopy, 270.
orrhorrhœa, 255.
orthopædia, 265.
orthopnœa, 265.
os, 110, 169.
oscheocele, 237.
oscheoplasty, 253.
ostalgia, 235.
osteitis, 241.
osteoblast, 265.
osteology, 244.
osteomalacia, 245.
osteoid, 248.
osteotomy, 260.
ostium, 159.

silica, 106.
sinapis, 112.
sine, 184.
sinister, 44.
singultus, 139.
sinus, 124.
-sis, 255.
sitis, 112.
situs, 124.
skeleton, 267.
skull, 298.
soda, 296.
solidus, 177.
solvus, 142.
somiferus, 177.
somnus, 128.
sopor, 108.
souffle, 292.
species, 126.
spectroscope, 270.
spectrum, 174.
speculum, 131.
spermatology, 244.
spermatorrhœa, 255.
spes, 126.
sphenoid, 248.
sphincter, 109.
sphygmograph, 238.
spigelia, 105.
spinalis, 181.
spiraculum, 131.
spiralis, 181.
spiritus, 45, 124.
splanchnocele, 235.
splanchnology, 244.
splenalgia, 235.
splenectomy, 235.
splenitis, 242.
splenomalacia, 245.
splenoncus, 250.
spondylitis, 242.
spurius, 177.
sputum, 174.
stamen, 174.
staphyloma, 250.
staphylitis, 242.
staphylorrhaphy, 253.
staphylotomy, 260.
statice, 97.
stavesacre, 33.
stear, 109.
steatoma, 250.
stercus, 185.

sternum, 174.
stertor, 109.
stibium, 174.
stigma, 119.
stethoscopy, 258.
stimulus, 128.
sthenic, 240.
stomachus, 248.
stomatitis, 242.
stomatocace, 236.
strabismus, 259.
stramonium, 177.
strangury, 261.
stratum, 177.
stria, 105.
styptic, 240.
suavis, 185.
sub, 184.
sublimatus, 177.
subsultus, 124.
subter, 184.
succedaneum, 177.
succinum, 177.
succus, 128.
sudor, 109.
sulcus, 128.
sulphur, 11.
sumach, 29.
sumbul, 29.
sunt, 99.
super, 184.
superficies, 126.
superus, 155.
supra, 183.
surdus, 177.
surgery, 13.
sutura, 105.
sycoma, 250.
symblepharon, 229.
symbol, 229.
symmetry, 229.
sympathy, 229.
symphysis, 229.
symptoma, 119.
symtomatology, 245.
synchysis, 229.
syncope, 229.
synchronous, 229.
syndesmitis, 242.
syndesmology, 245.
synechia, 229.
synovia, 229.
synthesis, 229.

syntonin, 229.
syphilis, 43.
syphilography, 238.
syphiliphobia, 252.
syringotomy, 261.
system, 229.
systole, 229.

T.

tabes, 174.
tabula, 110.
tache cerebrale, 292.
tactus, 124.
tænia, 110.
talipes, 188.
talis, 185.
talus, 134.
tamarind, 30.
tampon, 292.
tanacetum, 177.
tansy, 51.
tantus, 185.
tarantism, 41.
taraxacum, 30.
tarsus, 135.
taxis, 112.
tea, 32.
tegmen, 134.
temporalis, 185.
temperament, 10.
tempus, 177.
tenaculum, 131.
tener, 139.
tendo, 177.
tenesmus, 259.
tenontology, 245.
tenotomy, 261.
tepidus, 185.
teratology, 245.
terminus, 134.
tertianus, 185.
testes, 42, 112.
testudo, 177.
tetanoid, 248.
tetrad, 231.
tetrandrous, 231.
theca, 267.
thenar, 267.
theobroma, 42.
theomania, 246.
theopathy, 252.
therapeutics, 267.
thermalis, 185.

MEDICAL

AND

HYGIENIC WORKS

PUBLISHED BY

D. APPLETON & CO., 1, 3, & 5 Bond Street, New York.

BARKER (FORDYCE). On Sea-Sickness. A Popular Treatise for Travelers and the General Reader. Small 12mo. Cloth, 75 cents.

BARKER (FORDYCE). On Puerperal Disease. Clinical Lectures delivered at Bellevue Hospital. A Course of Lectures valuable alike to the Student and the Practitioner. Third edition. 8vo. Cloth, $5.00; sheep, $6.00.

BARTHOLOW (ROBERTS). A Treatise on Materia Medica and Therapeutics. **Sixth edition.** Revised, enlarged, and adapted to "The New Pharmacopœia." 8vo. Cloth, $5.00; sheep, $6.00.

BARTHOLOW (ROBERTS). A Treatise on the Practice of Medicine, for the Use of Students and Practitioners. **Sixth edition,** revised and enlarged. 8vo. Cloth, $5.00; sheep, $6.00.

BARTHOLOW (ROBERTS). On the Antagonism between Medicines and between Remedies and Diseases. Being the Cartwright Lectures for the Year 1880. 8vo. Cloth, $1.25.

BASTIAN (H. CHARLTON). Paralysis: Cerebral, Bulbar, and Spinal. Illustrated. Small 8vo. Cloth, $4.50.

BASTIAN (H. CHARLTON). The Brain as an Organ of the Mind. 12mo. Cloth, $2.50.

BELLEVUE AND CHARITY HOSPITAL REPORTS. Edited by W. A. Hammond, M. D. 8vo. Cloth, $4.00.

BENNET (J. H.). On the Treatment of Pulmonary Consumption, by Hygiene, Climate, and Medicine. Thin 8vo. Cloth, $1.50.

BILLINGS (F. S.). The Relation of Animal Diseases to the Public Health, and their Prevention. 8vo. Cloth, $4.00.

BILLROTH (THEODOR). General Surgical Pathology and Therapeutics. A Text-Book for Students and Physicians. Translated from the tenth German edition, by special permission of the author, by Charles E. Hackley, M. D. **Fifth American edition, revised and enlarged.** 8vo. Cloth, $5.00; sheep, $6.00.

BRAMWELL (BYROM). Diseases of the Heart and Thoracic Aorta. Illustrated with 226 Wood-Engravings and 68 Lithograph Plates—showing 91 Figures—in all 317 Illustrations. 8vo. Cloth, $8.00; sheep, $9.00.

BRYANT (JOSEPH D.). A Manual of Operative Surgery. **New edition, revised and enlarged.** 793 Illustrations. 8vo. Cloth, $5.00; sheep, $6.00.

BUCK (GURDON). Contributions to Reparative Surgery, showing its Application to the Treatment of Deformities produced by Destructive Disease or Injury; Congenital Defects from Arrest or Excess of Development; and Cicatricial Contractions following Burns. Illustrated by Thirty Cases and fine Engravings. 8vo. Cloth, $3.00.

CAMPBELL (F. R.). The Language of Medicine. A Manual giving the Origin. Etymology, Pronunciation, and Meaning of the Technical Terms found in Medical Literature. 8vo. (*In press.*)

CARPENTER (W. B.). Principles of Mental Physiology, with their Application to the Training and Discipline of the Mind, and the Study of its Morbid Conditions. 12mo. Cloth, $3.00.

CARTER (ALFRED H.). Elements of Practical Medicine. **Third edition,** revised and enlarged. 12mo. Cloth, $3.00.

CHAUVEAU (A.). The Comparative Anatomy of the Domesticated Animals. Translated and edited by George Fleming. Illustrated. 8vo. Cloth, $6.00.

COMBE (ANDREW). The Management of Infancy, Physiological and Moral. Revised and edited by Sir James Clark. 12mo. Cloth, $1.50.

COOLEY. Cyclopædia of Practical Receipts, and Collateral Information in the Arts, Manufactures, Professions, and Trades, including Medicine, Pharmacy, and Domestic Economy. Designed as a Comprehensive Supplement to the Pharmacopœia, and General Book of Reference for the Manufacturer, Tradesman, Amateur, and Heads of Families. **Sixth edition,** revised and partly rewritten by Richard V. Tuson. With Illustrations. 2 vols., 8vo. Cloth, $9.00.

CORNING (J. L.). Brain Exhaustion, with some Preliminary Considerations on Cerebral Dynamics. Crown 8vo. Cloth, $2.00.

CORNING (J. L.). Local Anæsthesia in General Medicine and Surgery. Being the Practical Application of the Author's Recent Discoveries. With Illustrations. Small 8vo. Cloth, $1.25.

ELLIOT (GEORGE T.). Obstetric Clinic: A Practical Contribution to the Study of Obstetrics and the Diseases of Women and Children. 8vo. Cloth, $4.50.

EVETZKY (ETIENNE). The Physiological and Therapeutical Action of Ergot. Being the Joseph Mather Smith Prize Essay for 1881. 8vo. Limp cloth, $1.00.

FLINT (AUSTIN). Medical Ethics and Etiquette. Commentaries on the National Code of Ethics. 12mo. Cloth, 60 cents.

FLINT (AUSTIN). Medicine of the Future. An Address prepared for the Annual Meeting of the British Medical Association in 1886. With Portrait of Dr. Flint. 12mo. Cloth, $1.00.

FLINT (AUSTIN, Jr.). Text-Book of Human Physiology; designed for the Use of Practitioners and Students of Medicine. Illustrated by three Lithographic Plates, and three hundred and thirteen Woodcuts. **Third edition, revised.** Imperial 8vo. Cloth, $6.00; sheep, $7.00.

FLINT (AUSTIN, Jr.). The Physiological Effects of Severe and Protracted Muscular Exercise; with Special Reference to its Influence upon the Excretion of Nitrogen. 12mo. Cloth, $1.00.

FLINT (AUSTIN, Jr.). Physiology of Man. Designed to represent the Existing State of Physiological Science as applied to the Functions of the Human Body. Complete in 5 vols., 8vo. Per vol., cloth, $4.50; sheep, $5.50.

*** Vols. I and II can be had in cloth and sheep binding; Vol. III in sheep only. Vol. IV is at present out of print.

3

FLINT (AUSTIN, Jr.). The Source of Muscular Power. Arguments and Conclusions drawn from Observation upon the Human Subject under Conditions of Rest and of Muscular Exercise. 12mo. Cloth, $1.00.

FLINT (AUSTIN, Jr.). Manual of Chemical Examinations of the Urine in Disease; with Brief Directions for the Examination of the most Common Varieties of Urinary Calculi. Revised edition. 12mo. Cloth, $1.00.

FOTHERGILL (J. MILNER). Diseases of Sedentary and Advanced Life. 8vo. Cloth, $2.00.

FOURNIER (ALFRED). Syphilis and Marriage. Translated by P. Albert Morrow, M. D. 8vo. Cloth, $2.00; sheep, $3.00.

FREY (HEINRICH). The Histology and Histochemistry of Man. A Treatise on the Elements of Composition and Structure of the Human Body. Translated from the fourth German edition by Arthur E. J. Barker, M. D., and revised by the author. With 608 Engravings on Wood. 8vo. Cloth, $5 00; sheep, $6.00.

FRIEDLANDER (CARL). The Use of the Microscope in Clinical and Pathological Examinations. Second edition, enlarged and improved, with a Chromo-lithograph Plate. Translated, with the permission of the author, by Henry C. Coe. M. D. 8vo. Cloth, $1.00.

GAMGEE (JOHN). Yellow Fever a Nautical Disease. Its Origin and Prevention. 8vo. Cloth, $1.50.

GARMANY (JASPER J.). Operative Surgery on the Cadaver. With Two Colored Diagrams showing the Collateral Circulation after Ligatures of Arteries of Arm, Abdomen, and Lower Extremity. Small 8vo. Cloth, $2.00.

GERSTER (ARPAD G.). The Rules of Aseptic and Antiseptic Surgery. A Practical Treatise for the Use of Students and the General Practitioner. Illustrated with over two hundred fine Engravings. 8vo. Cloth, $5.00; sheep, $6.00.

GROSS (SAMUEL W.). A Practical Treatise on Tumors of the Mammary Gland. Illustrated. 8vo. Cloth, $2.50.

GUTMANN (EDWARD). The Watering-Places and Mineral Springs of Germany, Austria, and Switzerland. Illustrated. 12mo. Cloth, $2.50.

GYNÆCOLOGICAL TRANSACTIONS. 8vo. Cloth, per volume, $5.00.

Vol. VIII. Being the Proceedings of the Eighth Annual Meeting of the American Gynaecological Society, held in Philadelphia, September 18, 19, and 20, 1883.

Vol. IX. Being the Proceedings of the Ninth Annual Meeting of the American Gynaecological Society, held in Chicago, September 30, and October 1 and 2, 1884.

Vol. X. Being the Proceedings of the Tenth Annual Meeting of the American Gynaecological Society, held in Washington, D. C., September 22, 23, and 24, 1885.

Vol. XI. Being the Proceedings of the Eleventh Annual Meeting of the American Gynaecological Society, held in Baltimore, Maryland, September, 21, 22, and 23, 1886

Vol. XII. Being the Proceedings of the Twelfth Annual Meeting of the American Gynaecological Society, held in New York, Tuesday, Wednesday, and Thursday, September 13, 14, and 15, 1887.

HAMMOND (W. A.). A Treatise on Diseases of the Nervous System. **Eighth edition,** rewritten, enlarged, and improved. 8vo. Cloth, $5.00; sheep, $6.00.

HAMMOND (W. A.). A Treatise on Insanity, in its Medical Relations. 8vo. Cloth, $5.00; sheep, $6.00.

HAMMOND (W. A.). Clinical Lectures on Diseases of the Nervous System. Delivered at Bellevue Hospital Medical College. Edited by T. M. B. Cross, M. D. 8vo. Cloth, $3.50.

HARVEY (A.). First Lines of Therapeutics. 12mo. Cloth, $1.50.

HOFFMANN–ULTZMANN. Analysis of the Urine, with Special Reference to Diseases of the Urinary Apparatus. By M. B. Hoffmann, Professor in the University of Gratz; and R. Ultzmann, Tutor in the University of Vienna. **Second enlarged and improved edition.** 8vo. Cloth, $2.00.

HOWE (JOSEPH W.). Emergencies, and how to treat them. Fourth edition, revised. 8vo. Cloth, $2.50.

HOWE (JOSEPH W.). The Breath, and the Diseases which give it a Fetid Odor. With Directions for Treatment. **Second edition,** revised and corrected. 12mo. Cloth, $1.00.

HUEPPE (FERDINAND). The Methods of Bacteriological Investigation. Written at the request of Dr. Robert Koch. Translated by Hermann M. Biggs, M. D. Illustrated. 8vo. Cloth, $2.50.

HUXLEY (T. H.). The Anatomy of Vertebrated Animals. Illustrated. 12mo. Cloth, $2.50.

HUXLEY (THOMAS HENRY). The Anatomy of Invertebrated Animals. Illustrated. 12mo. Cloth, $2.50.

JACCOUD (S.). The Curability and Treatment of Pulmonary Phthisis. Translated and edited by Montagu Lubbock, M. D. 8vo. Cloth, $4.00.

JONES (H. MACNAUGHTON). Practical Manual of Diseases of Women and Uterine Therapeutics. For Students and Practitioners. 188 Illustrations. 12mo. Cloth, $3.00.

KEYES (E. L.). A Practical Treatise on Genito-Urinary Diseases, including Syphilis. Being a new edition of a work with the same title, by Van Buren and Keyes. Almost entirely rewritten. 8vo. With Illustrations. Cloth, $5.00; sheep, $6.00.

KEYES (E. L.). The Tonic Treatment of Syphilis, including Local Treatment of Lesions. 8vo. Cloth, $1.00.

KINGSLEY (N. W.). A Treatise on Oral Deformities as a Branch of Mechanical Surgery. With over 350 Illustrations. 8vo. Cloth, $5.00; sheep, $6.00.

LEGG (J. WICKHAM). On the Bile, Jaundice, and Bilious Diseases. With Illustrations in Chromo-Lithography. 8vo. Cloth, $6.00; sheep, $7.00.

LITTLE (W. J.). Medical and Surgical Aspects of In-Knee (Genu-Valgum): its Relation to Rickets, its Prevention, and its Treatment, with and without Surgical Operation. Illustrated by upward of Fifty Figures and Diagrams. 8vo. Cloth, $2.00.

LORING (EDWARD G.). A Text-Book of Ophthalmoscopy. Part I. The Normal Eye, Determination of Refraction, and Diseases of the Media. With 131 Illustrations, and 4 Chromo-Lithographs. 8vo. Cloth, $5.00.

LUSK (WILLIAM T.). The Science and Art of Midwifery. With 246 Illustrations. **Second edition, revised and enlarged.** 8vo. Cloth, $5.00; sheep, $6.00.

LUYS (J.). The Brain and its Functions. With Illustrations. 12mo. Cloth, $1.50.

MARKOE (T. M.). A Treatise on Diseases of the Bones. With Illustrations. 8vo. Cloth, $4.50.

MAUDSLEY (HENRY). Body and Mind: an Inquiry into their Connection and Mutual Influence, specially in reference to Mental Disorders. An enlarged and revised edition, to which are added Psychological Essays. 12mo. Cloth, $1.50.

MAUDSLEY (HENRY). Physiology of the Mind. Being the first part of a third edition, revised, enlarged, and in great part rewritten, of "The Physiology and Pathology of the Mind." 12mo. Cloth, $2.00.

MAUDSLEY (HENRY). Pathology of the Mind. Third edition. 12mo. Cloth, $2.00.

MAUDSLEY (HENRY). Responsibility in Mental Disease. 12mo. Cloth, $1.50.

NEFTEL (WM. B.). Galvano-Therapeutics. The Physiological and Therapeutical Action of the Galvanic Current upon the Acoustic, Optic, Sympathetic, and Pneumogastric Nerves. 12mo. Cloth, $1.50.

NEUMANN (ISIDOR). Hand-Book of Skin Diseases. Translated by Lucius D. Bulkley, M.D. Illustrated by 66 Wood-Engravings. 8vo. Cloth, $4.00; sheep, $5.00.

THE NEW YORK MEDICAL JOURNAL (weekly). Edited by Frank P. Foster, M.D. Terms per annum, $5.00.
Binding Cases, cloth, 50 cents each.
GENERAL INDEX, from April, 1865, to June, 1876 (23 vols.) 8vo. Cloth, 75 cents.

NIEMEYER (FELIX VON). A Text-Book of Practical Medicine, with particular reference to Physiology and Pathological Anatomy. Containing all the author's Additions and Revisions in the eighth and last German edition. Translated by George H. Humphreys, M.D., and Charles E. Hackley, M.D. 2 vols., 8vo. Cloth, $9.00; sheep, $11.00.

NIGHTINGALE'S (FLORENCE) Notes on Nursing. 12mo. Cloth, 75 cents.

PEASLEE (E. R.). A Treatise on Ovarian Tumors: their Pathology, Diagnosis, and Treatment, with reference especially to Ovariotomy. With Illustrations. 8vo. Cloth, $5.00; sheep, $6.00.

PEREIRA'S (Dr.) Elements of Materia Medica and Therapeutics. Abridged and adapted for the Use of Medical and Pharmaceutical Practitioners and Students, and comprising all the Medicines of the British Pharmacopœia, with such others as are frequently ordered in Prescriptions, or required by the Physician. Edited by Robert Bentley and Theophilus Redwood. Royal 8vo. Cloth, $7.00; sheep, $8.00.

PEYER (ALEXANDER). An Atlas of Clinical Microscopy. Translated and edited by Alfred C. Girard, M.D. First American, from the manuscript of the second German edition, with Additions. Ninety Plates, with 105 Illustrations, Chromo-Lithographs. Square 8vo. Cloth, $6.00.

POMEROY (OREN D.). The Diagnosis and Treatment of Diseases of the Ear. With One Hundred Illustrations. **Second edition,** revised and enlarged. 8vo. Cloth, $3.00.

POORE (C. T.). Osteotomy and Osteoclasis, for the Correction of Deformities of the Lower Limbs. 50 Illustrations. 8vo. Cloth, $2.50.

QUAIN (RICHARD). A Dictionary of Medicine, including General Pathology, General Therapeutics, Hygiene, and the Diseases peculiar to Women and Children. By Various Writers. Edited by Richard Quain, M. D., In one large 8vo volume, with complete Index, and 138 Illustrations. (*Sold only by subscription.*) Half morocco, $8.00.

RANNEY (AMBROSE L.). Applied Anatomy of the Nervous System, being a Study of this Portion of the Human Body from a Standpoint of its General Interest and Practical Utility, designed for Use as a Text-Book and as a Work of Reference. Profusely illustrated. 8vo. Cloth, $4.00; sheep, $5.00.

RANNEY (AMBROSE L.). Lectures on Electricity in Medicine, delivered at the Medical Department of the University of Vermont, Burlington. Numerous Illustrations. 12mo. Cloth, $1.00.

RANNEY (AMBROSE L.). Practical Suggestions respecting the Varieties of Electric Currents and the Uses of Electricity in Medicine, with Hints relating to the Selection and Care of Electrical Apparatus. With Illustrations and 14 Plates. 16mo. Cloth, $1.00.

RIBOT (TH.). Diseases of Memory: an Essay in the Positive Psychology. Translated from the French by William Huntington. 12mo. Cloth, $1.50.

RICHARDSON (B. W.). Diseases of Modern Life. 12mo. Cloth, $2.00.

RICHARDSON (B. W.). A Ministry of Health and other Addresses. 12mo. Cloth, $1.50.

ROBINSON (A. R.). A Manual of Dermatology. Revised and corrected. 8vo. Cloth, $5.00.

ROSCOE SCHORLEMMER. Treatise on Chemistry.
    Vol. 1. Non-Metallic Elements. 8vo. Cloth, $5.00.
    Vol. 2. Part 1. Metals. 8vo. Cloth, $3.00.
    Vol 2. Part II. Metals. 8vo. Cloth, $3.00.
    Vol. 3. Part I. The Chemistry of the Hydrocarbons and their Derivatives. 8vo. Cloth, $5.00.
    Vol. 3. Part II. The Chemistry of the Hydrocarbons and their Derivatives. 8vo. Cloth, $5.00.
    Vol. 3. Part III. This part commences the consideration of the complicated but most important series of bodies known as the Aromatic Compounds. 8vo. Cloth, $3.00.

ROSENTHAL (I.). General Physiology of Muscles and Nerves. With 75 Woodcuts. 12mo. Cloth, $1.50.

SAYRE (LEWIS A.). Practical Manual of the Treatment of Club-Foot. **Fourth edition, enlarged and corrected.** 12mo. Cloth, $1.25.

SAYRE (LEWIS A.). Lectures on Orthopedic Surgery and Diseases of the Joints, delivered at Bellevue Hospital Medical College. **New edition,** illustrated with 324 Engravings on Wood. 8vo. Cloth, $5.00; sheep, $6.00.

SCHROEDER (KARL). A Manual of Midwifery, including the Pathology of Pregnancy and the Puerperal State. Translated into English from the third German edition, by Charles H. Carter, M. D. With 26 Engravings on Wood. 8vo. Cloth, $3.50; sheep, $4.50.

SHOEMAKER (JOHN V.). A Text-Book of Diseases of the Skin. Six Chromo-Lithographs and numerous Engravings. 8vo. Cloth, $5.00; sheep, $6.00.

SIMPSON (JAMES Y.). Selected Works: Anæsthesia, Diseases of Women. 3 vols., 8vo. Per volume. Cloth, $3.00; sheep, $4.00.

SKENE (ALEXANDER J. C.) A Text-Book on the Diseases of Women. 8vo. Illustrated with over two hundred fine Engravings. (In press.)

SMITH (EDWARD). Foods. 12mo. Cloth, $1.75.

SMITH (EDWARD). Health: A Hand-Book for Households and Schools. Illustrated. 12mo. Cloth, $1.00.

STEINER (JOHANNES). Compendium of Children's Diseases: a Hand-Book for Practitioners and Students. Translated from the second German edition, by Lawson Tait. 8vo. Cloth, $3.50; sheep, $4.50.

STEVENS (GEORGE T) Functional Nervous Diseases: their Causes and their Treatment. Memoir for the Concourse of 1881–1883, Académie Royal de Médecine de Belgique. With a Supplement, on the Anomalies of Refraction and Accommodation of the Eye, and of the Ocular Muscles. Small 8vo. With six Photographic Plates and twelve Illustrations. Cloth, $2.50.

STONE (R. FRENCH). Elements of Modern Medicine, including Principles of Pathology and of Therapeutics, with many Useful Memoranda and Valuable Tables of Reference. Accompanied by Pocket Fever Charts. Designed for the Use of Students and Practitioners of Medicine. In wallet-book form, with pockets on each cover for Memoranda, Temperature Charts, etc. Roan, tuck, $2.50.

STRECKER (ADOLPH). Short Text-Book of Organic Chemistry. By Dr. Johannes Wislicenus. Translated and edited, with Extensive Additions, by W. H. Hodgkinson and A. J. Greenaway. 8vo. Cloth, $5.00.

STRÜMPELL (ADOLPH). A Text-Book of Medicine, for Students and Practitioners. With 111 Illustrations. 8vo. Cloth, $6.00; sheep, $7.00.

SWANZY (HENRY R.). A Hand-Book of the Diseases of the Eye, and their Treatment. With 122 Illustrations, and Holmgren's Tests for Color-Blindness. Crown 8vo. Cloth, $3.00.

TRACY (ROGER S.). The Essentials of Anatomy, Physiology, and Hygiene. 12mo. Cloth, $1.25.

TRACY (ROGER S.). Hand-Book of Sanitary Information for Householders. Containing Facts and Suggestions about Ventilation, Drainage, Care of Contagious Diseases, Disinfection, Food, and Water. With Appendices on Disinfectants and Plumbers' Materials. 16mo. Cloth, 50 cents.

TRANSACTIONS OF THE AMERICAN LARYNGOLOGICAL ASSOCIATION. 8vo. Cloth, $2.50 per volume.

 Vol. V. Being the Proceedings of the Sixth Annual Meeting, held in the city of New York, May 12, 13, and 14, 1884.

 Vol. VI. Being the Proceedings of the Seventh Annual Meeting, held in Detroit, June 24, 25, and 26, 1885.

TRANSACTIONS OF THE NEW YORK STATE MEDICAL ASSOCIA-TION, VOL. I. Being the Proceedings of the First Annual Meeting of the New York State Medical Association, held in New York, November 18, 19, and 20, 1884. Small 8vo. Cloth, $5.00.

TYNDALL (JOHN). Essays on the Floating Matter of the Air, in Relation to Putrefaction and Infection. 12mo. Cloth, $1.50.

ULTZMANN (ROBERT). Pyuria, or Pus in the Urine, and its Treatment Translated by permission, by Dr. Walter B. Platt. 12mo. · Cloth, $1.00.

VAN BUREN (W. H.). Lectures upon Diseases of the Rectum, and the Surgery of the Lower Bowel, delivered at Bellevue Hospital Medical College. **Second edition, revised and enlarged.** 8vo. Cloth, $3.00; sheep, $4.00.

VAN BUREN (W. H.). Lectures on the Principles and Practice of Surgery. Delivered at Bellevue Hospital Medical College. Edited by Lewis A. Stimson, M. D. 8vo. Cloth, $4.00; sheep, $5.00.

VOGEL (A.). A Practical Treatise on the Diseases of Children. Translated and edited by H. Raphael, M. D. **Third American from the eighth German edition, revised and enlarged.** Illustrated by six Lithographic Plates. 8vo. Cloth, $4.50; sheep, $5.50.

VON ZEISSL (HERMANN). Outlines of the Pathology and Treatment of Syphilis and Allied Venereal Diseases. **Second edition,** revised by Maximilian von Zeissl. Authorized edition. Translated, with Notes, by H. Raphael, M. D. 8vo. Cloth, $4.00; sheep, $5.00.

WAGNER (RUDOLF). Hand-Book of Chemical Technology. Translated and edited from the eighth German edition, with extensive Additions, by William Crookes. With 336 Illustrations. 8vo. Cloth, $5.00.

WALTON (GEORGE E.). Mineral Springs of the United States and Canadas. Containing the latest Analyses, with full Description of Localities, Routes, etc. **Second edition, revised and enlarged.** 12mo. Cloth, $2.00.

WEBBER (S. G.). A Treatise on Nervous Diseases: Their Symptoms and Treatment. A Text-Book for Students and Practitioners. 8vo. Cloth, $3.00.

WEEKS (CLARA S.). A Text-Book of Nursing. For the Use of Training-Schools, Families, and Private Students. 12mo. With 13 Illustrations, Questions for Review and Examination, and Vocabulary of Medical Terms. 12mo. Cloth, $1.75.

WELLS (T. SPENCER). Diseases of the Ovaries. 8vo. Cloth, $4.50.

WYETH (JOHN A.). A Text-Book on Surgery: General, Operative, and Mechanical. Profusely illustrated. (*Sold by subscription only.*) 8vo. Buckram, uncut edges, $7.00; sheep, $8.00; half morocco, $8.50.

WYLIE (WILLIAM G.). Hospitals: Their History, Organization, and Construction. 8vo. Cloth, $2.50.

www.ingramcontent.com/pod-product-compliance
Lightning Source LLC
Chambersburg PA
CBHW021119270326
41929CB00009B/949